Mast Cell Disorders

Editor

CEM AKIN

IMMUNOLOGY AND ALLERGY CLINICS OF NORTH AMERICA

www.immunology.theclinics.com

Consulting Editor
ROHIT KATIAL

November 2023 • Volume 43 • Number 4

ELSEVIER

1600 John F. Kennedy Boulevard • Suite 1800 • Philadelphia, Pennsylvania, 19103-2899
http://www.theclinics.com

IMMUNOLOGY AND ALLERGY CLINICS OF NORTH AMERICA Volume 43, Number 4

November 2023 ISSN 0889-8561, ISBN-13: 978-0-443-18183-2

Editor: Taylor Hayes
Developmental Editor: Nitesh Barthwal

Immunology and Allergy Clinics of North America (ISSN 0889–8561) is published quarterly by Elsevier Inc., 360 Park Avenue South, New York, NY 10010-1710. Months of issue are February, May, August, and November. Periodicals postage paid at New York, NY and additional mailing offices. Subscription prices are $365.00 per year for US individuals, $704.00 per year for US institutions, $100.00 per year for US students and residents, $445.00 per year for Canadian individuals, $100.00 per year for Canadian students, $895.00 per year for Canadian institutions, $470.00 per year for international individuals, $895.00 per year for international institutions, $220.00 per year for international students. To receive student/resident rate, orders must be accompanied by name of affiliated institution, date of term, and the *signature* of program/residency coordinator on institution letterhead. Orders will be billed at individual rate until proof of status is received. Foreign air speed delivery is included in all *Clinics* subscription prices. All prices are subject to change without notice. **POSTMASTER:** Send address changes to *Immunology and Allergy Clinics of North America,* Elsevier Health Sciences Division, Subscription Customer Service, 3251 Riverport Lane, Maryland Heights, MO 63043. **Customer Service: 1-800-654-2452 (U.S. and Canada); 314-447-8871 (outside U.S. and Canada). Fax: 314-447-8029. E-mail: journalscustomerservice-usa@elsevier.com** (for print support); **journalsonlinesupport-usa@elsevier.com** (for online support).

Reprints. For copies of 100 or more, of articles in this publication, please contact the Commercial Reprints Department, Elsevier Inc., 360 Park Avenue South, New York, New York 10010-1710. Tel. 212-633-3874, Fax: 212-633-3820, E-mail: reprints@elsevier.com.

Immunology and Allergy Clinics of North America is covered in MEDLINE/PubMed (Index Medicus), Current Contents/Life Sciences, Science Citation Index, ISI/BIOMED, Chemical Abstracts, and EMBASE/Excerpta Medica.

Contributors

CONSULTING EDITOR

ROHIT KATIAL, MD, FAAAAI, FACAAI, FACP
Professor of Medicine, Associate Vice President of Education, Director, Center for Clinical Immunology, Irene J. & Dr. Abraham E. Goldminz, Chair in Immunology and Respiratory Medicine, Division of Allergy and Clinical Immunology, Department of Medicine, National Jewish Health, University of Colorado, Denver, Colorado, USA

EDITOR

CEM AKIN, MD, PhD
Professor of Medicine, Division of Allergy and Clinical Immunology, University of Michigan, Ann Arbor, Michigan, USA

AUTHORS

CEM AKIN, MD, PhD
Professor of Medicine, Division of Allergy and Clinical Immunology, University of Michigan, Ann Arbor, Michigan, USA

MICHEL AROCK, PharmD, PhD
Department of Hematological Biology, Pitie-Salpetriere Hospital, Platform of Molecular Analysis for Mastocytosis and Mast Cell Activation Syndromes (MCAS), Saint-Antoine Hospital, DMU BioGem, AP-HP, Sorbonne University, Paris, France

MARIANA C. CASTELLS, MD, PhD
Professor, Division of Allergy and Clinical Immunology, Brigham and Women's Hospital, Harvard Medical School, Boston, Massachusetts, USA

GEORGE H. CAUGHEY, MD
Emeritus Professor of Medicine, University of California, San Francisco, San Francisco, California, USA

YANNICK CHANTRAN, PharmD, PhD
Department of Biological Hematology, Platform of Molecular Analysis for Mastocytosis and Mast Cell Activation Syndromes (MCAS), Pitie-Salpetriere Hospital, Department of Biological Immunology, Saint-Antoine Hospital, DMU BioGem, AP-HP, Sorbonne University, Health Environmental Risk Assessment (HERA) Team, Center of Research in Epidemiology and Statistics (CRESS), Inserm/INRAE, Faculty of Pharmacy, University of Paris, Paris, France

MICHAEL W. DEININGER, MD, PhD
Professor and Chief Scientific Officer, Versiti Blood Research Institute, Division of Hematology and Oncology, Medical College of Wisconsin, Milwaukee, Wisconsin, USA

SARA S. ELLINGWOOD, MD
Division of Allergy and Clinical Immunology, University of Michigan, Ann Arbor, Michigan, USA

ANDREW ESPELAND, BS, BA
Division of Allergy and Clinical Immunology, Brigham and Women's Hospital, Boston, Massachusetts, USA

MATTHEW P. GIANNETTI, MD
Allergy & Immunology Specialist, Division of Allergy and Clinical Immunology, Brigham and Women's Hospital, Harvard Medical School, Boston, Massachusetts, USA

GRACE GODWIN, BA
Division of Allergy and Clinical Immunology, Brigham and Women's Hospital, Boston, Massachusetts, USA

THEO GULEN MD, PhD
Senior Consultant Allergist, Department of Respiratory Medicine and Allergy, Division of Immunology and Allergy, Department of Medicine Solna, Karolinska Institutet, Mastocytosis Centre Karolinska, Karolinska University Hospital Huddinge, Stockholm, Sweden

MATTHEW J. HAMILTON, MD
Lead Gastroenterologist, Mastocytosis Center, Brigham and Women's Hospital, Crohn's and Colitis Center, Assistant Professor of Medicine, Harvard Medical School, Chestnut Hill, Massachusetts, USA

HANS-PETER HORNY, MD
Institute of Pathology, Paracelsus Medical University, Salzburg, Austria, Institute of Pathology, Ludwig Maximilian University, Munich, Germany

NINELA IRGA-JAWORSKA, MD, PhD
Assistant Professor, Department of Pediatrics, Hematology and Oncology, Medical University of Gdansk, Gdansk, Poland

ANNA KOVALSZKI, MD, FAAAAI
Associate Professor of Medicine, Division of Allergy and Clinical Immunology, University of Michigan, Ann Arbor, Michigan, USA

MAGDALENA LANGE, MD, PhD
Professor, Department of Dermatology, Venerology and Allergology, Medical University of Gdansk, Gdansk, Poland

JULIA MIDDLESWORTH, BS
Clinical Research Coordinator, Division of Allergy and Clinical Immunology, Brigham and Women's Hospital, Boston, Massachusetts, USA

JENNIFER NICOLORO-SANTABARBARA, PhD
Instructor of Psychiatry, Harvard Medical School, Department of Psychiatry, Brigham and Women's Hospital, Boston, Massachusetts, USA

POLINA PYATILOVA, MD
Institute of Allergy, Charité – Berlin University Medicine, Corporate Member of Freie Berlin University Medicine and Humboldt University of Berlin, Fraunhofer Institute for Translational Medicine and Pharmacology, Immunology and Allergy, Berlin, Germany

JOANNA RENKE, MD, PhD
Assistant Professor, Department of Pediatrics, Hematology and Oncology, Medical University of Gdansk, Gdansk, Poland

FRANK SIEBENHAAR, MD
Institute of Allergy, Charité – Berlin University Medicine, Corporate Member of Freie Univeristy of Berlin and Humboldt University of Berlin, Fraunhofer Institute for Translational Medicine and Pharmacology, Immunology and Allergy, Berlin, Germany

KARL SOTLAR, MD
Head, Institute of Pathology, Paracelsus Medical University, Salzburg, Austria

TSEWANG TASHI, MD
Assistant Professor, Division of Hematology and Hematologic Malignancies, Huntsman Cancer Institute, University of Utah, Salt Lake City, Utah, USA

PETER VALENT, MD
Austrian hematologist, Division of Hematology and Hemostaseology, Department of Internal Medicine I, Ludwig Boltzmann Institute for Hematology and Oncology, Medical University of Vienna, Town, Austria

Contents

Experts of the European Competence Network on Mastocytosis (ECNM) and the American Initiative on Mast Cell Disorders have discussed and updated diagnostic criteria and the classification of mastocytosis, based on new insights in the field and data collected in recent years, mostly within ECNM registry projects in which studies on several thousand cases have been performed. Based on this proposal, the World Health Organization has updated its classification of mastocytosis. This article discusses the revised classification of mastocytosis in light of a rapidly moving field and the advent of new diagnostic parameters, new prognostication tools, and new therapies.

A *KIT* activating mutation (usually *KIT* D816V) is detected in neoplastic cells in greater than 90% of indolent patients with systemic mastocytosis (SM). In more advanced variants of SM, additional genetic defects can be found in several myeloid malignancy-related genes, which can be detected by applying next-generation sequencing. Currently, the techniques recommended to detect the *KIT* D816V mutation and quantify the mutational burden in peripheral blood, bone marrow, or other organs/tissues are allele specific-quantitative PCR or droplet digital PCR. These techniques are useful for diagnosis, prognostication, follow-up and monitoring of therapeutic efficacy of cytoreductive agents in patients with SM.

To a large extent, the clinical picture of pediatric mastocytosis depends on the age at which it is diagnosed. A neonate with diffuse cutaneous mastocytosis may frequently present in a severe state requiring treatment. Toddlers may require long-term anti-mediator therapy, and this may lead to concerns such as organizing preschool education due to the need for epinephrine injections. A teenager may have to face cutaneous disease persistence or a diagnosis of systemic mastocytosis. Further studies are needed to refine the available treatment options and prognosis for different age groups.

Mastocytosis is characterized by expansion and activation of clonally aberrant mast cells (MCs) in one or more organ systems. Inappropriate MC activation is a key finding in both allergy and mastocytosis; therefore, symptoms in both conditions show some degree of overlap. When mediator release is excessive and involves multiple systems, anaphylaxis may occur. In mastocytosis, the prevalence of atopy is similar to those of the general population, whereas the incidence of anaphylaxis is significantly higher. The purpose of this review is to discuss features of allergy and anaphylaxis as well as the principles of managing MC mediator release symptoms in mastocytosis.

Patients with mastocytosis have an increased risk for mast cell activation events including anaphylaxis when exposed to certain drugs and Hymenoptera venom. Hypotension and cardiovascular collapse without skin or other systemic manifestations can occur after Hymenoptera stings, during the perioperative period, and after exposure to nonsteroidal ntiinflammatory drugs, opioids, and other mast cell activating medications, including vancomycin and quinolones. This chapter reviews the epidemiology, mechanisms, diagnosis, management, and treatment options for Hymenoptera venom and drug-induced reactions in patients with mastocytosis.

Gastrointestinal symptoms are prevalent in patients with systemic mastocytosis and contribute to morbidity. In indolent disease, the symptoms, which include heartburn, abdominal pain, and diarrhea, are largely due to release of mast cell mediators but may be due to other factors. A thorough evaluation that incorporates abdominal imaging and endoscopy with intestinal biopsy assists with diagnosis and management. Patients with advanced mastocytosis experience signs and symptoms of gastrointestinal dysfunction owing to the massive infiltration of clonal mast cells in the tissues. The gastrointestinal symptoms in systemic mastocytosis are treatable with a combination of therapies, including those directed at mast cells.

Advanced systemic mastocytosis (AdvSM) is a heterogeneous group of disorders characterized by neoplastic mast cell-related organ damage and frequently associated with a myeloid neoplasm. The 3 clinical entities that comprise AdvSM are aggressive SM (ASM), SM-associated hematologic neoplasm, and mast cell leukemia. A gain-of-function KIT D816 V mutation is the primary oncogenic driver found in about 90% of all patients with AdvSM. Midostaurin, an oral multikinase inhibitor with activity against KIT D816V, and avapritinib, an oral selective KIT D816V inhibitor are approved for AdvSM.

Systemic mastocytosis is associated with KIT D816V mutation in more than 90% of cases. Patients with non-advanced forms of mastocytosis (indolent systemic mastocytosis, bone marrow mastocytosis, and smoldering systenic mastocytosis) have a low rate of progession to advanced variants and generally have a comparable life expectancy to age-matched general population. Symptomatology in non-advanced mastocytosis is variable and is related to mast cell mediator release. While some patients require no or minimal symptomatic therapy with antimediator drugs, other may suffer from refractory symptoms impacting the quality of life despite being on multiple anti-mediator drugs. KIT tyrosine kinase inhibitors have been approved for advanced SM, and avapritinib has also been recently approved as the first such inhibitor for indolent systemic mastocytosis. Other TKIs are currently in clinical trials for patients with non-advanced SM who have persistent and severe symptoms despite optimized antimediator therapy. This article will review the current state of the science and available clinical data from trials of tyrosine kinase inhibitors in non-advanced systemic mastocytosis.

Mastocytosis is a heterogeneous disease with a wide spectrum of signs, symptoms, and concomitant disorders, such as skin lesions, anaphylaxis, osteoporosis, gastrointestinal involvement, and organomegaly. Disease specificity for frequently reported symptoms, such as fatigue, headache, anxiety, and brain fog, is poorly defined and need to be addressed in further studies. Patients with CM and non-AdvSM are mostly affected by mast cell mediator–related symptoms, whereas in AdvSM symptoms also result from organ damage, which makes their assessment challenging. In this paper we discuss approaches currently used to measure symptom burden and QoL impairment in relation to the clinical phenotype.

This article reviews the effects of gender on anaphylaxis in general and focuses on mastocytosis-specific issues. Incidence of anaphylaxis is increased in female compared with male patients during the pubertal years through the fifth decade of life, in which these differences decrease. Estrogen is thought to increase the severity of anaphylaxis through increased endothelial nitric oxide synthase release. Despite this, all-cause fatal anaphylaxis does not appear to show a gender predilection. Systemic mastocytosis incidence is higher in women; however, mortality is increased in men owing to increased molecular and cytogenetic abnormalities.

Mast cell granules are packed with proteases, which are released with other mediators by degranulating stimuli. Several of these proteases are targets of potentially therapeutic inhibitors based on hypothesized contributions to diseases, notably asthma and ulcerative colitis for β-tryptases, heart and kidney scarring for chymases, and airway infection for dipeptidyl peptidase-I. Small-molecule and antibody-based β-tryptase inhibitors showing preclinical promise were tested in early-phase human trials with some evidence of benefit. Chymase inhibitors were given safely in Phase II trials without demonstrating benefits, whereas dipeptidyl peptidase-I inhibitor improved bronchiectasis, in effects likely related to inactivation of the enzyme in neutrophils.

IMMUNOLOGY AND ALLERGY CLINICS OF NORTH AMERICA

SERIES OF RELATED INTEREST

Medical Clinics
https://www.medical.theclinics.com/

THE CLINICS ARE AVAILABLE ONLINE!
Access your subscription at:
www.theclinics.com

Foreword
Mast Cell Disorders

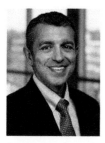

Rohit Katial, MD, FAAAAI, FACAAI, FACP
Consulting Editor

Mast cell disorders are a relatively rare and heterogenous group of diseases but increasingly are being recognized as our understanding of mast cell biology continues to grow. The spectrum of mast cell disease can cause a variety of symptoms ranging from benign to malignant potential. Such diseases were previously seen primarily in the hematology therapeutic area. However, scientific advancement in the understanding of the pathophysiology of mast cell diseases, ranging from increased gene copy number to hyperreleasability, has placed the allergist and immunologist in the center of managing such conditions. As a result, classification schemes of these disorders has also evolved over time. In parallel, drug development has accelerated with less toxic options having recently been approved for indolent systemic mastocytosis, and others are in late-stage development. Dr Cem Aiken has assembled a world-class set of authors to provide an overview of the current knowledge and research on mast cell disorders, as well as practical guidance for health care professionals. Review topics ranging from mast cell biology, classification of disorders, to management with special emphasis on gender as well as a focus on gastrointestinal manifestations are reflected in this comprehensive issue of the *Immunology and Allergy Clinics of North America*. I highly recommend this issue both as a knowledge update and as future reference when treating patients with suspected mast cell problems.

Rohit Katial, MD, FAAAAI, FACAAI, FACP
Center for Clinical Immunology
National Jewish Health
University of Colorado
Denver, CO, USA

E-mail address:
KatialR@NJHealth.org

Immunol Allergy Clin N Am 43 (2023) xiii
https://doi.org/10.1016/j.iac.2023.08.001
0889-8561/23/© 2023 Published by Elsevier Inc.

Preface

Mastocytosis: Aiming for the Right Targets

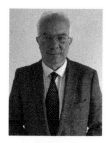

Cem Akin, MD, PhD
Editor

We have witnessed important and historic developments in mastocytosis in the last year. Diagnostic criteria and classification of mastocytosis have been revised by the World Health Organization and International Consensus Classification groups. FDA approved avapritinib for the treatment of indolent systemic mastocytosis, the first cyto-reductive targeted therapy with selectivity against D816V KIT mutation. Availability of new drugs made us think harder about coming up with symptom scores and quality-of-life measures to document response to therapies. Taken together, these developments will change the way we diagnose, classify, and treat mastocytosis in the years to come. Therefore, this issue of the *Immunology and Allergy Clinics of North America* is timely and aims to provide the reader with an update directly from the experts who have been involved in these advancements. I am grateful to each of the authors who contributed their time and expertise to this collection.

The issue begins with an expert overview by Dr Valent and colleagues of the most recent changes in classification and diagnostic criteria of mastocytosis. In the next article, Dr Arock and Dr Chantran review KIT mutations, which are crucial to understand the rationale for new targeted therapy options. Dr Renke and colleagues discuss pediatric and hereditary mastocytosis, which still remains to be better understood in their pathogenesis and treatment options. Next, Dr Gulen provides an overview of management of mediator-related symptoms, as these symptoms are experienced by most patients regardless of their disease category. Dr Castells and colleagues provide specific guidance about drug and venom allergies, two of the most concerning allergic comorbidities in mastocytosis. Gastrointestinal symptoms are commonly experienced by patients, and their management may be challenging, often requiring partnership with a gastroenterologist experienced in the field, such as Dr Hamilton, who reviews the state-of-the-art. Patients with advanced mastocytosis often have

Immunol Allergy Clin N Am 43 (2023) xv–xvi
https://doi.org/10.1016/j.iac.2023.06.001
0889-8561/23/© 2023 Published by Elsevier Inc.

immunology.theclinics.com

complex disease pathogenesis with associated myeloid neoplasms or organ dysfunction due to massive mast cell infiltration and require management by Hematologists. Dr Tashi and Dr Deininger share the guiding principles of management of these challenging disease variants, which have been revolutionized by the availability of D816V KIT targeting tyrosine kinase inhibitors. On the indolent disease front, things have been anything but quiet. While patients with nonadvanced disease generally have a low rate of progression and histopathologically stable disease burden, many suffer from recurrent mast cell activation symptoms despite being on optimized antimediator therapies. The next article reviews the use of tyrosine kinase inhibitors, including Avapritinib, a selective D816V KIT tyrosine kinase inhibitor, which has become the first cytoreductive drug approved by the FDA on May 22, 2023, for treatment of indolent disease. Such availability of cytoreductive therapies as well as other emerging drug candidates for treatment of indolent disease underscored the necessity of development of tools of assessment of disease burden and quality of life to identify patients who are candidates for these therapies as well as assess to response to them. Dr Pyatilova and Dr Siebenhaar's article provides an excellent comparative review of these assessment tools. The next article, by Dr Ellingwood and Dr Kovalszki, is rather unique in its perspective on focusing on gender differences in mastocytosis as well as anaphylaxis. Finally, the issue concludes with a discussion by Dr Caughey, on mast cell proteases and their therapeutic targeting.

Mastocytosis is a rare but underdiagnosed disease. I often hear from patients about the value of connecting with an expert to make the appropriate diagnosis and institute the right treatment. The American Initiative on Mastocytosis was recently established to promote research and close the knowledge gap between the referral centers and the general community of providers and patients (aimcd.net). I sincerely hope that this issue of the *Immunology and Allergy Clinics of North America* contributes to this aim.

Cem Akin, MD, PhD
University of Michigan
24 Frank Lloyd Wright Drive
PO Box 442, Suite H-2100
Ann Arbor, MI 48106, USA

E-mail address:
cemakin@umich.edu

World Health Organization Classification and Diagnosis of Mastocytosis

Update 2023 and Future Perspectives

Peter Valent, MD[a],*, Karl Sotlar, MD[b], Hans-Peter Horny, MD[b,c], Michel Arock, PharmD, PhD[d,e], Cem Akin, MD[f]

KEYWORDS

• Mast cells • Mastocytosis • Diagnostic criteria • WHO classification • ICC

KEY POINTS

- Over the past few years, a number of new diagnostic and prognostic markers relevant to mast cell neoplasms and/or mast cell activation disorders have been identified.
- Based on these markers, the ECNM/AIM consensus group has proposed updated diagnostic criteria and an updated classification of mastocytosis and mast cell activation syndromes.
- The World Health Organization and International Consensus Classification (ICC) have adopted this proposal and introduced updates with slight modifications.

INTRODUCTION AND HISTORICAL BACKGROUND

Mast cells (MC) are multifunctional cells of the immune system that reside in the connective tissues and mucosal sites in various organs.[1–5] In common with blood basophils, MC produce and store a number of proinflammatory and immune-regulatory mediators in their metachromatic granules, including histamine, heparin, tryptases, cytokines, and chemokines.[1–5] MC also express numerous cell surface receptors, including complement-binding sites, cytokine receptors, and the high-affinity receptor for IgE, also known as FcεRI.[1–7] During activation by an external ligand, such as an

[a] Division of Hematology and Hemostaseology, Department of Internal Medicine I, Ludwig Boltzmann Institute for Hematology and Oncology, Medical University of Vienna, Wäheringer Gürtel 18-20, A-1090 Vienna, Austria; [b] Institute of Pathology, Paracelsus Medical University Salzburg, Austria; [c] Institute of Pathology, Ludwig Maximilians University, Munich, Germany; [d] Department of Hematological Biology, Pitié-Salpêtrière Hospital, DMU BioGem, AP-HP. Sorbonne University, Paris, France; [e] Platform of Molecular Analysis for Mastocytosis and Mast Cell Activation Syndromes (MCAS), Saint-Antoine Hospital, DMU BioGem, AP-HP. Sorbonne University, Paris, France; [f] Division of Allergy and Clinical Immunology, University of Michigan, Ann Arbor, MI, USA
* Corresponding author.
E-mail address: peter.valent@meduniwien.ac.at

Immunol Allergy Clin N Am 43 (2023) 627–649
https://doi.org/10.1016/j.iac.2023.04.011
0889-8561/23/© 2023 Elsevier Inc. All rights reserved.

allergen or complement components, MC release their granular mediators into the extracellular space. In addition, during activation, MC synthesize and release newly formed membrane-derived lipid mediators, cytokines, and chemokines.[1–7]

Mastocytosis is a group of hematologic disorders characterized by an expansion and accumulation of clonal MC in the skin, bone marrow (BM), and/or other internal organs, such as the liver, spleen, or gastrointestinal (GI) tract.[1,3,4,8–12] Based on the typical (pigmented) skin lesions and local response to rubbing or scratching, mastocytosis was first described as an unusual form of urticaria by Nettleship and Tay in 1869.[13] Some years later, the name urticaria pigmentosa (UP) was coined, and following Paul Ehrlich's description of MC in 1879[14], the presence and accumulation of MC in UP lesions was reported by Unna in 1887.[15] For several decades, mastocytosis was considered to be a disease limited to the skin. However, in 1949, Ellis reported on a case with systemic mastocytosis (SM) in an autopsy section.[16] Over time, SM has become a well-recognized disease, whereas other patients reportedly have UP without systemic involvement. These patients, most of them children, are diagnosed with cutaneous mastocytosis (CM), which has an excellent prognosis.[8–12] A localized benign variant of CM, termed mastocytoma of skin, has also been described.[10–12]

In general, the basic concept of splitting mastocytosis into CM and SM remains valid. However, during the past 30 years, several clinically and prognostic distinct subtypes of CM and SM have been identified.[17–20] Between 1990 and 2000, several specific markers of SM were reported and used to coin a set of diagnostic criteria.[21–30] These criteria were discussed by experts from Europe and the United States in the Year 2000 Working Conference on Mastocytosis and used to establish a solid classification of the disease,[31] which was adopted by the World Health Organization (WHO) in 2001[32] and was updated and reconfirmed in 2008, 2016, and 2022.[33–38]

Based on WHO criteria, SM is divided into bone marrow mastocytosis (BMM), indolent SM (ISM), smoldering SM (SSM), aggressive SM (ASM), SM with an associated hematopoietic neoplasm (SM-AHN), and MC leukemia (MCL).[31–38] In most patients with SM, the disease-triggering *KIT* D816V mutation is identified in neoplastic cells.[9,10,18,22–25] The prognosis and course of SM varies among patients, depending on the disease variant, clinical and molecular features, and patient-associated variables. Regarding progression and survival, an important factor is the presence of a concomitant myeloid neoplasm, such as chronic myelomonocytic leukemia (CMML), myelodysplastic syndromes, myeloproliferative neoplasms, or acute myeloid leukemia (AML).[18,29,31–35] In these patients, neoplastic cells often exhibit chromosomal abnormalities and additional somatic mutations in critical (driver) genes, like *TET2*, *SRSF2*, *ASXL1*, *JAK2*, *RUNX1*, or *RAS*.[39–48] The prognosis in these patients is usually poor and dictated by the aggressiveness of the detected AHN.

In the past 15 years, several additional prognostic disease features have been identified and validated in patients with SM. Moreover, multiparameter score systems have been developed in which overall and progression-free survival can now be better predicted.[46,49–51] Furthermore, new treatment concepts have been established in the recent past, such as KIT D816V-targeting tyrosine kinase inhibitors, allogeneic hematopoietic stem cell transplantation, immunotherapies, and IgE-targeting approaches.[35,36,52–61] These treatments have greatly improved the prognosis, survival, and quality of life in patients with SM.[52–61]

However, in the past few years, additional disease-related parameters and genetic lesions have been identified. In addition, patients with mastocytosis may suffer from mediator-related symptoms, which may be severe despite therapy. In those with severe and recurrent symptoms of anaphylaxis, an MC activation syndrome (MCAS) may be diagnosed.[62–65]

A genetic condition potentially influencing the severity and frequency of mediator-related symptoms in SM is hereditary alpha-tryptasemia (HαT). In fact, HαT is an autosomal dominant trait defined by an enhanced copy number of the *TPSAB1* gene encoding alpha-tryptase.[66–69] Most carriers of HαT have an elevated basal serum tryptase level. Patients with SM who carry HαT also have higher tryptase levels (as one would expect from MC numbers recorded in tissue sections) and may suffer from recurrent severe anaphylaxis and MCAS, especially when a concomitant allergy is also present.[68,69] Indeed, IgE-dependent allergies are relevant comorbidities in SM.[3,52,69–74]

This article provides an update of diagnostic criteria and the classification of MC disorders in light of novel developments in the field, new markers and prognostic scores, and new drugs and treatment options for patients with advanced SM.

REVIEW AND DISCUSSION OF THE CURRENT CLASSIFICATION OF MC DISORDERS

The following paragraphs present and discuss the refined diagnostic criteria and the updated classification of mastocytosis as presented by an international consensus group, the WHO, and the International Consensus Classification (ICC) consortium. In addition, the global classification of MC disorders as well as the criteria and classification of MCAS proposed by the consensus group are discussed.

UPDATED WHO CLASSIFICATION OF MASTOCYTOSIS 2022

As mentioned before, the WHO classification of mastocytosis was established in 2001 and refined in 2008, 2016, and 2022. To assist the WHO, a consensus group consisting of experts from Europe and the United States organized working conferences to discuss new developments in the field and related updates and refinements in diagnostic criteria in 2000,[31] 2005,[75] 2010,[62] 2012,[10] 2015,[12,35] and 2020.[37] The updated criteria and classification of mastocytosis proposed by this consensus group in 2021[37] were again adopted with slight modifications by the WHO in 2022.[38] Based on the current WHO classification, mastocytosis is divided into CM, BMM, ISM, SSM, SM-AHN, ASM, MCL, and MC sarcoma (**Table 1**). Extracutaneous mastocytoma is also recognized as a separate type of mastocytosis.[37,38] However, based on its rarity, this disease is usually not listed in published tables among MC disorders in the WHO classification.[37,38] Nevertheless, to provide a complete spectrum of disorders, this rare entity has been included in **Table 1**.

The WHO has also mentioned the well-differentiated morphology of MC as an important morphologic feature in SM.[37,38] However, a well-differentiated MC morphology in SM is rare and can occur in any type of SM. In the well-differentiated subtypes of SM, neoplastic MC usually lack CD25 and *KIT* D816V (MC may express other KIT mutant forms in such cases), which has diagnostic implications and may be associated with sensitivity against imatinib.[76–79] The diagnostic criteria and classification of mastocytosis proposed by the consensus group was also adopted with slight modifications by a second expert panel (ICC group) in 2022.[80] In all these proposals, the basic concept to classify mastocytosis and the basic criteria that have been developed and provided by the consensus group between 2000 and 2022[12,31,37,62,75] remain essentially unchanged.

CUTANEOUS MASTOCYTOSIS VERSUS SKIN INVOLVEMENT IN SM

In most childhood patients with mastocytosis, CM is diagnosed.[9–12] By contrast, CM is only rarely diagnosed in adulthood. Rather, most adult patients with cutaneous lesions are suffering from SM but not from CM.[9–12,31] Therefore, in adult patients, a BM

Table 1
World Health Organization classification of mastocytosis

Variant Subvariant	Abbreviation
Cutaneous mastocytosis	CM
Maculopapular CM	MPCM
(Urticaria pigmentosa)[a]	UP[a]
Diffuse CM	DCM
Mastocytoma of skin	-
Systemic mastocytosis[b]	SM
Bone marrow mastocytosis	BMM
Indolent SM	ISM
Smoldering SM	SSM
SM with and associated hematologic neoplasm	SM-AHN
Aggressive SM	ASM
Mast cell leukemia	MCL
Mast cell sarcoma	MCS
Extracutaneous mastocytoma[c]	-

[a] The term *urticaria pigmentosa* (UP) is still in use and is still regarded standard, but should be replaced by the term MPCM.
[b] In a few patients with SM, mast cells are rather mature and well granulated. In these cases, a well-differentiated subtype of SM (SM_{WD}) can be diagnosed. This SM_{WD} type may be found in any WHO variant of SM.
[c] Extracutaneous mastocytoma is a very rare nonmalignant disease variant that has mostly been reported in lung tissue. Based on its rarity this variant is not listed in the current classifications of mastocytosis.[35,37,38]

investigation is always recommended, whereas in children, a BM is usually not performed unless clear signs for a systemic advanced disease are present.[9–12,35,75,81,82] In children, CM is defined by typical skin lesions, a positive Darier sign, and the absence of clinical signs of systemic involvement.[11] In adults, CM is defined by typical skin lesions, the Darier sign and/or a positive skin histology, and, most importantly, absence of criteria sufficient to diagnose SM (**Table 2**).[9–12,31,83]

The discrimination between CM and SM in adults is of prognostic significance, because patients with CM have a more favorable outcome regarding survival.[83] Another important point is that in patients with CM, systemic involvement with clonal MC and 1 or 2 minor SM criteria are not sufficient for the diagnosis of SM. Rather, SM can only be diagnosed when at least 1 major and 1 minor or at least 3 minor SM criteria are met.[9–12,31–35] In adults with skin lesions without histologic staging (no BM studies available), the provisional diagnosis of "mastocytosis in the skin" (MIS) is appropriate.[11,12,31,37] In children, the provisional diagnosis of MIS is not applied unless basal serum tryptase levels exceed 100 ng/mL and signs for an advanced SM or other myeloid neoplasm are present.[11,12,35] Otherwise, the diagnosis in children is CM even without a BM investigation.

Once diagnosed, CM should be subclassified into maculopapular CM (MPCM), diffuse CM, and cutaneous mastocytoma (see **Table 2**).[9–12,31–35,37] Diagnostic criteria for CM subsets are listed in **Table 2**. Most children with CM and almost all adults with CM or SM exhibit maculopapular lesions. In most of the children, skin lesions fade and disappear before or during puberty. Two prognostic subtypes of childhood MPCM can be delineated: a variant characterized by monomorphic, small-sized skin lesions and a second form defined by polymorphic (often larger) lesions (see **Table 2**).[11,37,83,84] The monomorphic skin pattern is also found in adults with CM or SM, suggesting that such

Table 2
Classification and typical features (criteria) of cutaneous mastocytosis and cutaneous involvement in SM

Variant and Subvariants	Abbreviation	Features/Criteria
A. Maculopapular cutaneous mastocytosis	MPCM	Positive Darier sign[a]
		Typical pigmented skin lesions
		Positive histology[b]
		KIT mutation in lesional skin
(1) Monomorphic variant	MPCM-m	Monomorphic skin lesions[c]
		Criteria for SM not fulfilled[d]
(2) Polymorphic variant	MPCM-p	Polymorphic skin lesions[c]
		Criteria for SM not fulfilled[d]
B. Diffuse cutaneous mastocytosis	DCM	Positive Darier sign[a]
		Diffuse involvement of the entire skin
		Positive histology[b]
		Criteria for SM not fulfilled[d]
C. Cutaneous mastocytoma	-	Positive Darier sign[a]
		Positive histology[b]
(1) Isolated mastocytoma		1 single lesion
(2) Multilocalized mastocytomas		2 or 3 lesions
		Criteria for SM not fulfilled[d]
D. Cutaneous involvement in SM[e]		Criteria for SM fulfilled

[a] The Darier sign and the typical skin lesions are major diagnostic criteria. A positive histology and the presence of an activating KIT mutation are minor diagnostic criteria. In patients with atypical lesions or a negative Darier sign, the diagnosis of mastocytosis can still be established provided that minor criteria are fulfilled. Testing for the Darier sign should always be done gently and only when needed for diagnosis.

[b] Histologic examination includes standard stains and immunohistochemistry using antibodies against tryptase and KIT regardless of the variant (monomorphic or polymorphic). The numbers of KIT+/tryptase+ mast cells are usually increased in skin lesions in patients with mastocytosis.

[c] The monomorphic variant is found in children and adults. When found in children, the likelihood that the lesions persist into adulthood is high. Polymorphic skin lesions are detected in childhood MPCM but usually not in adults. When detected in children, the likelihood that these polymorphic lesions disappear later during or after puberty in adolescence is relatively high.[11]

[d] In all adult patients, SM has to be excluded by staging investigations including bone marrow studies. In children, bone marrow studies are only performed when clinical signs and symptoms are indicative of an advanced hematologic disease.

[e] Usually seen in adults; almost all of these patients present with monomorphic skin lesions.

Adapted from Valent P, Akin C, Hartmann K, et al. Updated diagnostic criteria and classification of mast cell disorders: a consensus proposal. Hemasphere. 2021;5(11):e646; with permission.

skin lesions may persist into adulthood (with or without progression to SM), whereas polymorphic skin lesions usually disappear.[11,83,84] Therefore, childhood MPCM should further be split (subclassified) into a monomorphic and a polymorphic type (see **Table 2**).[11,37,83]

MAJOR AND MINOR CRITERIA TO DIAGNOSE SM: UPDATE 2023

According to the basic definition established in 2000 by the consensus group, the diagnosis of SM is made when at least 1 major and 1 minor or at least 3 minor SM criteria are fulfilled (**Table 3**).[10,12,31–35] Major SM criterion is the multifocal infiltration of internal (extracutaneous) organs (usually BM) by MC forming compact aggregates (clusters) of at least 15 MC (see **Table 3**).[31–35] In some of the patients, MC infiltrates may be masked or distorted by an AHN. In such cases, the diagnosis of SM (finally

Table 3
Major and minor diagnostic criteria of systemic mastocytosis (SM)

Major criterion	Multifocal dense infiltrates of mast cells (>15 mast cells in aggregates) in bone marrow biopsies and/or in sections of other extracutaneous organs
Minor criteria	1. >25% of all mast cells are atypical cells (type I or type II) on bone marrow smears or are spindle-shaped in mast cell infiltrates detected in sections of BM or other extracutaneous organs[a]
	2. KIT-activating *KIT* point mutations at codon 816 or in other critical regions of *KIT*[b] in bone marrow or another extracutaneous organ
	3. Mast cells in bone marrow, blood, or another extracutaneous organ express one or more of: CD2, CD25, and/or CD30[c]
	4. Baseline serum tryptase concentration >20 ng/mL (in the case of an unrelated myeloid neoplasm, an elevated tryptase level does not count as an SM criterion; in the case of a known hereditary HαT, the tryptase level should be adjusted[d]).
	If at least 1 major and 2 minor *or* 3 minor criteria are fulfilled → the diagnosis is SM

[a] In tissue sections, an abnormal mast cell morphology counts in both a compact infiltrate and a diffuse (or mixed diffuse + compact) mast cell infiltrate. However, the spindle-shaped form does not count as an SM criterion when mast cells are lining vascular cells, fat cells, nerve cells, or the endosteal-lining cell layer. In the bone marrow smear, an atypical morphology of mast cells does not count as SM criterion when mast cells are located in or adjacent to the bone marrow particles. Morphologic criteria of atypical mast cells have been described.[28]
[b] Any type of *KIT* mutation counts as minor SM criterion when published solid evidence for its transforming behavior is available.
[c] All 3 markers fulfill this minor SM criterion when expression can be confirmed by flow cytometry, immunohistochemistry, or both techniques.
[d] Although the optimal way of adjustment may still need to be defined, one way is to divide the basal tryptase level by 1 plus the extra copy numbers of the alpha-tryptase gene. Example: when the tryptase level is 30 and 2 extra copies of the alpha-tryptase gene are found in a patient with HαT, the HαT-corrected tryptase level is 10 (30/3 = 10) and thus is not a minor SM criterion.
Adapted from Valent P, Akin C, Hartmann K, et al. Updated diagnostic criteria and classification of mast cell disorders: a consensus proposal. Hemasphere. 2021;5(11):e646; with permission.

SM-AHN) can often only be established by demonstrating 3 minor SM criteria or after successful cytoreductive therapy was applied.

An abnormal morphology of MC, usually in the form of spindle-shaped hypogranulated cells, serves as the first minor SM criterion (see **Table 3**).[31–35,37] At least 25% of MC in BM smears or histologies must display these features to qualify as minor SM criterion.[31–35] Even if only a diffuse MC infiltration is found without compact MC aggregates, the abnormal MC morphology (≥25%) counts as a minor SM criterion.[37] On the other hand, it is important to know that the spindle-shaped morphology does not count for MC that are lining blood vessels, nerves, fat cells, or the endosteal surface layer.[31,35,37,75]

Aberrant expression of CD2, CD25, and/or CD30 in/on MC serves as a phenotypic minor criterion of SM (see **Table 3**).[37] All 3 markers are applicable in multicolor flow cytometry (usually in the BM) and in tissue sections (mostly BM) by immunohistochemistry. In daily practice, tryptase, CD25, and CD30 are usually applied (**Fig. 1**). CD2 and CD25 were defined as minor SM criterion since 2001,[31] whereas the expression of CD30 has now been added as an additional minor SM criterion in 2020.[37] Indeed, CD30 expression in MC is completely specific for SM, but is not found in other myeloid neoplasms.[85–88] On the other hand, CD30 is not expressed in MC in all patients with SM

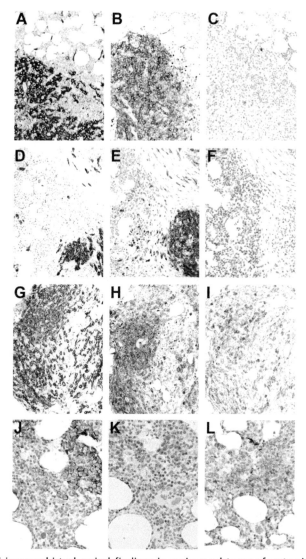

Fig. 1. Typical immunohistochemical findings in various subtypes of systemic mastocytosis (SM). (*A–C*) a compact MC infiltrate in the bone marrow of a patient with indolent SM (ISM) stained with antibodies against KIT (CD117) (*A*), CD25 (*B*), and CD30 (*C*). (*D–F*), in another patient with ISM, mast cells not only expressed CD117 (*D*) and CD25 (*E*), but did also express some CD30 (*F*). *G–I*, in a case of SM-AHN (ASM-MDS/MPN), besides expression of CD117 (*G*) and CD25 (*H*), most mast cells were also found to strongly display CD30 (*I*). *J–L*, in a patients with SM with well-differentiated morphology (SMWD) (*J*), mast cells typically express KIT (CD117) (*J*) but lack CD25 (*K*). However, aberrant expression of CD30 (*L*) confirms the neoplastic nature of mast cells and thus the diagnosis of SM.

(see **Fig. 1**). According to published data, CD30 is detectable in neoplastic MC in most cases with ISM and advanced SM by flow cytometry and/or immunohistochemistry.[85–88] A major advantage of CD30 (over CD2 and CD25) is that this antigen is also displayed by MC in patients with SM with a well-differentiated morphology (SM_WD), where MC often lack CD2 and CD25 (see **Fig. 1**)[87]; this is important because these patients may otherwise not fulfill any other minor SM criterion even if the major criterion is met. Initially CD30 expression in MC was also reported to correlate roughly with a more advanced phase/type of SM.[85] However, subsequent validation did not confirm this correlation.[88] Therefore, CD30 is not recommended as a grading marker in SM.

Several *KIT* variants may be detected in neoplastic cells in SM.[22–25,76–78,89–91] The most frequently detected variant is D816V.[22–25,89–92] This *KIT* mutation is detected in approximately 90% of all adult patients with ISM and SSM and most with SM-AHN.[22–25,89,92] Other activating mutations in *KIT* are by far less frequent and may be identified in cases with childhood mastocytosis and in adults with advanced SM or SM$_{WD}$.[76–78,89–92] According to the latest update of the consensus group and the WHO as well as the ICC, any activating mutation in *KIT* counts as minor SM criterion.[37,38,80] In some patients with MCL and in true mast cell sarcoma (MCS) (without signs of SM), neoplastic cells may lack *KIT* D816V and other *KIT* mutations.

Patients with SM typically present with an increased basal serum tryptase concentration.[9,10,12,21,29–35] As per the consensus group proposal, a clearly elevated basal serum tryptase level ($\geq$20 ng/mL) counts as a minor SM criterion.[31–35,37,62,75] It is important to know that elevated tryptase levels may also be recorded in other conditions and pathologies, such as an AHN, kidney (renal) failure, allergic (anaphylactic) reactions, and HαT.[31–35,66–69] As a result, several restrictions have to be taken into account in clinical practice: (1) only the *basal* serum tryptase level obtained in a symptom-free interval qualifies as a minor SM criterion, (2) tryptase does not count as criterion when an AHN is present, and (3) in patients with known HαT, the tryptase level should be adjusted by dividing the basal tryptase concentrations by one plus the extra copy numbers of *TPSAB1*. However, the polymerase chain reaction (PCR) test measuring *TPSAB1* copies is not generally available (not even in all mastocytosis centers). In patients with unknown *TPSAB1* status, the old definition of this SM criterion must be applied in clinical practice.

DIAGNOSTIC CRITERIA FOR BONE MARROW MASTOCYTOSIS (BMM) AND SEPARATION FROM OTHER SM VARIANTS

Until 2020, BMM was a provisional subvariant of ISM (ISM without skin lesions) in the proposal of the consensus group and in the WHO classification.[31–35] However, recent studies have shown that patients with BMM with low disease burden (defined as no B-finding and a tryptase level <125 ng/mL) have a better prognosis than patients with typical ISM or SSM.[93]

It is also essential to separate BMM from advanced SM and aleukemic MCL where skin lesions are also often absent.[31–35] According to the most recent proposal of the consensus group, which also forms the basis of the WHO classification, BMM is defined as a separate SM variant without skin lesions, in which no (not a single) B-finding is recorded and basal serum tryptase is less than 125 ng/mL.[37,93] As soon as 1 single B-finding is identified and/or serum tryptase exceeds 125 ng/mL, the diagnosis changes from BMM to ISM without skin lesions[37]; this is also the case when diagnostic MC infiltrates are found in an extramedullary organ. However, in most patients with BMM, MC infiltrates are small sized even in the BM, so that the diagnosis depends on 3 documented minor SM criteria. A summary of the diagnostic criteria for BMM, typical ISM (with or without skin lesions), and SSM is shown in **Table 4**.

Additional clinical features of BMM are relatively frequent and often severe (IgE-dependent) allergic reactions, especially to bee and/or wasp venom (often resulting

Table 4
Proposed revised criteria for bone marrow mastocytosis (BMM), typical indolent systemic mastocytosis (ISM), ISM without skin involvement, and smoldering systemic mastocytosis (SSM)

Variant	Criteria
BMM	SM criteria fulfilled
	No skin lesions
	No B-findings
	No C-findings
	Basal serum tryptase level <125 ng/mL
	No dense SM infiltrates in an extramedullary organ
	No signs/criteria for MCL
	No signs/criteria for an AHN
(Typical) ISM	SM criteria fulfilled
	Typical skin lesions
	No or one B-finding
	No C-finding
	No signs/criteria for MCL
	No signs/criteria for an AHN
ISM without skin lesions	SM criteria fulfilled
	No skin lesions
	No or 1 B-finding[a] and/or basal serum tryptase level ≥125 ng/mL and/or dense SM infiltrates in an extramedullary organ
	No C-finding
	No signs/criteria for MCL
	No signs/criteria for an AHN
SSM	SM criteria fulfilled
	Two or three B-findings
	No C-finding
	No signs/criteria for MCL
	No signs/criteria for an AHN[b]

Abbreviation: VAF, variant allele frequency.
[a] Serum tryptase levels may exceed 200 ng/mL (if no other B-finding is detected) or be less than 200 ng/mL (in which case one B-finding may be detected).
[b] Additional mutations in other (driver) genes, such as *TET2*, may be detected by next-generation sequencing (NGS). However, when new gene variants occur or the VAF increases over time, a re-examination of the bone marrow is required to exclude SM-AHN.
Adapted from Valent P, Akin C, Hartmann K, et al. Updated diagnostic criteria and classification of mast cell disorders: a consensus proposal. Hemasphere. 2021;5(11):e646; with permission.

in MCAS) and osteoporosis. In most of the patients, *KIT* D816V is detected in BM samples. However, in a few cases, especially those with a well-differentiated MC morphology, no mutation in *KIT* at codon 816 is found. The prognosis of BMM regarding progression into advanced SM is favorable, although some patients may develop an AHN.[93]

UPDATED FORMULATION OF B-FINDINGS AND C-FINDINGS

In the delineation between BMM, ISM, SSM, and ASM or MCL, it is crucial to ask for the presence of B-findings and C-findings, which are depicted in **Box 1**. As mentioned, the presence of 2 or 3 B-findings and the absence of C-findings is consistent with the diagnosis of SSM.[12,17,31–35,37] As soon as one or more C-findings are recorded, the patient has ASM, unless additional features and criteria are indicative of (A)SM-AHN or MCL (**Box 1**).[12,31–35,37]

Box 1
Role of B-findings and C-findings in the definition of bone marrow mastocytosis (BMM), indolent systemic mastocytosis (ISM), smoldering systemic mastocytosis (SSM), and aggressive systemic mastocytosis (ASM) or mast cell leukemia (MCL)

Number of B-findings	Number of C-findings	Potential Diagnosis[a]
0	0	BMM or ISM
1	0	ISM
2–3	0	SSM
0–3	1 or more[b]	ASM or MCL[a]

[a]In patients with 1 or more C-findings, the final diagnosis may be ASM, but may also be (A)SM-AHN or MCL. [b]Depending on the organ systems involved, patients with ASM or MCL may exhibit multiple C-findings.

B-findings define a high MC burden and disease expansion into various myeloid lineages and organ systems.[31–35,37] In contrast to C-findings, however, B-findings are not associated with organ damage. C-findings, in turn, are indicative of a clinically relevant SM-induced organ damage.[31–35,37] It is important to understand that the impact of SM on organ damage must be confirmed by demonstrating (by histology) that the local SM infiltrate is the underlying cause.[12,35,37] In cases with SM-AHN, it may be difficult to define the relative impact of SM and of the concomitant AHN, especially when both are advanced malignancies. In these patients, both disorders may cause organ damage.

B-findings and C-findings are shown in **Table 5**. The three B-findings include (1) direct indication of a huge number of neoplastic MC (*KIT*-mutated cells), (2) evidence of dysplasia or myeloproliferation (not meeting criteria of an AHN), and (3) organomegaly (lymphadenopathy, hepatomegaly, splenomegaly) (**Table 5**). The first B-finding is documented by a markedly increased serum tryptase level ($\geq$200 ng/mL) and/or a huge infiltration of the BM with neoplastic MC ($\geq$30%) as determined by immunohistochemistry. With regard to tryptase, it is important to correct the basal serum level by dividing by the total copy numbers of alpha-tryptase gene (see **Table 5**). In the latest update of the consensus proposal, one additional disease-related feature is now recognized as a B-finding, namely, a high variant allele frequency (VAF) of *KIT* D816V in aspirated BM cells or peripheral blood (PB) leukocytes (>10%) (see **Table 5**). B-findings may also be accompanied by major blood count abnormalities, such as leukocytosis (neutrophilia, monocytosis, or eosinophilia) or thrombocytosis, whereas severe cytopenia is a C-finding (but not a B-finding).

C-findings include severe persistent cytopenia (anemia, neutropenia, thrombocytopenia), malabsorption with hypoalbuminemia and weight loss, splenomegaly with massive hypersplenism, hepatopathy with massive ascites and elevated liver enzymes (including typically an increase in alkaline phosphatase), and large (often painful) osteolysis ($\geq$2 cm in diameter) with pathologic fractures (see **Table 5**). Weight loss per se is not regarded as a C-finding, and the same holds true for splenomegaly, hepatomegaly, or small-sized osteolyses.

UPDATED CRITERIA OF SMOLDERING SYSTEMIC MASTOCYTOSIS

In general, the definition and criteria applied to diagnose SSM have not changed over the past 20 years. In particular, SSM can be diagnosed when SM criteria are fulfilled,

Table 5
Proposed refined B-findings and C-findings

B-findings	C-findings (SM-induced Organ Damage)
High MC burden:	
Infiltration grade (MC) in BM ≥ 30% in histology (IHC) and/or serum tryptase level ≥200 ng/mL[a] and/or *KIT* D816V VAF ≥10% in BM or PB leukocytes	*Cytopenia*
	ANC < 1 × 10⁹/L
Signs of myeloproliferation and/or myelodysplasia[b]:	Hb < 10 g/dL
Hypercellular BM with loss of fat cells and prominent myelopoiesis ± left shift and eosinophilia ± leukocytosis and eosinophilia and/or discrete signs of myelodysplasia (<10% neutrophils, erythrocytes, and megakaryocytes)	PLT < 100 × 10⁹/L (1 or more found)
Organomegaly:	*Hepatopathy:*
Palpable hepatomegaly without ascites or other signs of organ damage and/or	Ascites and elevated liver enzymes[c] ± hepatomegaly or cirrhotic liver ± portal hypertension
palpable splenomegaly without hypersplenism and without weight loss and/or and lymphadenopathy	*Spleen:*
	Palpable splenomegaly with hypersplenism ± weight loss ± hypoalbuminemia
Palpable or visceral LN enlargement found in ULS or CT (>2 cm)	*GI tract:*
	Malabsorption with hypoalbuminemia ± weight loss
	Bone:
	Large-sized osteolysis (≥2 cm) with pathologic fracture ± bone pain

Abbreviations: ANC, absolute neutrophil count; BM, bone marrow; CT, computed tomography; Hb, hemoglobin; IHC, immunohistochemistry; LN, lymph node; MDS, myelodysplastic syndrome; MPN, myeloproliferative neoplasm; PB, peripheral blood; PLT, platelet count; ULS, ultrasound; VAF, variant allele frequency.

[a] In the case of a known HαT, the basal serum tryptase level should be adjusted. Although the optimal way of adjustment still needs to be defined, one way is to divide the basal tryptase level by 1 plus the extra copy numbers of the alpha-tryptase gene. Example: when the tryptase level is 300 and 2 extra copies of the alpha-tryptase gene are found in a patient with HαT, the HαT-corrected tryptase level is 100 (300/3 = 100) and would thus not qualify as a B-finding.

[b] Signs of myeloproliferation and/or myelodysplasia must be discrete and stable (neither disappear nor progress) and must not reach diagnostic criteria of an MPN, MDS, or MPN/MDS in which case the diagnosis changes to SM-AHN. The presence of a myeloid AHN excludes B-findings and SSM by definition.

[c] Alkaline phosphatase levels are typically elevated in patients with advanced SM and SM-induced liver damage. In some of these patients, only elevated levels of liver enzymes but no (clinically relevant) ascites is found.

Adapted from Valent P, Akin C, Hartmann K, et al. Updated diagnostic criteria and classification of mast cell disorders: a consensus proposal. Hemasphere. 2021;5(11):e646; with permission.

2 or 3 B-findings (but not a single C-finding) have been identified, and no signs/criteria for an AHN or MCL are detected (**Table 4**).[17,31–35,37] The revised B-findings outlined previously should be applied in each case to diagnose SSM.[37] As mentioned before, it is important to correct the serum tryptase level in all patients with HαT and suspected SSM.[37] It is also important to understand that SSM has a less favorable prognosis compared with patients with BMM or ISM regarding hematologic progression.[37,49,94] Therefore, patients with SSM should be followed carefully to detect signs of progression as early as possible. Useful follow-up parameters include serum tryptase levels, *KIT* D816V (VAF), and alkaline phosphatase. Most importantly, these patients are checked for progression of B-findings and development of C-findings, which changes the diagnosis from SSM to advanced SM (eg, ASM).[37,75]

REFINED CRITERIA FOR ASM AND ASM VARIANTS

A diagnosis of ASM can be established when SM criteria are met, at least one C-finding has been documented, and no signs/criteria indicative of an AHN or MCL are present.[10,12,31–35,37] Based on the proposal of the consensus group, ASM can be split into classical ASM (MC in BM smears <5%) and ASM in transformation to MCL (MC in BM smears ranging between 5% and 19%) (**Table 6**).[35,37,95] Furthermore, ASM cases can be split into those with pure ASM and those with ASM-AHN (see **Table 6**).[35,37,95] Finally, patients with ASM can be divided into those with primary ASM and those with secondary ASM developing from a less-advanced MC disease (see **Table 6**).[37,95] Despite more effective available therapies, patients with ASM may still progress to MCL or ASM-AHN. In these patients, intensive chemotherapy and hematopoietic stem cell transplantation have to be considered.[36,53]

SM-AHN AND AHN VARIANTS: STATUS 2023

Most AHN are myeloid neoplasms, whereas lymphoid AHN are very rare.[37,49,96] In each case, the AHN must be diagnosed using the WHO or ICC criteria. As per the consensus group proposal and the WHO, any type of a hematologic neoplasm qualifies as an AHN, including myeloid and lymphoid neoplasms, provided that the same organs are involved.[31–38] By contrast, the ICC only classifies (accepts) myeloid neoplasms as being directly associated with SM.[80] As a result, the ICC also proposed to change the term AHN (SM-AHN) into "associated myeloid neoplasms" (AMN) (SM-AMN).[80]

REFINEMENTS IN THE DIAGNOSIS OF MCL AND MAST CELL SARCOMA (MCS)

The basic definition and diagnostic criteria for MCL that have been formulated and refined by the consensus group and WHO between 2000 and 2020 remain essentially unchanged.[10,12,31–37,75,95] This basic proposal divides MCL into a classical, "leukemic" variant (MC ≥ 10% of all leukocytes in blood smears) and a more prevalent "aleukemic" form, known as aleukemic MCL (MC <10% in PB).[31,35,37,95] MCL can also be split into primary MCL (no preceding SM known) and secondary MCL following a previous (lower grade) SM, or MCS (see **Table 5**).[95] Moreover, patients with MCL can be divided into those with acute MCL (C-findings detectable) and those with chronic MCL without detectable C-findings (see **Table 5**).[95] Compared with acute MCL, patients with chronic MCL have a better prognosis and may show an excellent response to therapy with novel KIT-targeting drugs. However, in many of these

Table 6
Refined classification of advanced systemic mastocytosis (SM), including SM with an associated hematologic neoplasm (SM-AHN), aggressive SM (ASM), and mast cell leukemia

Category	Subvariant	Defining Key Features (Criteria)
SM-AHN	According to SM variant:	
	BMM-AHN	WHO criteria (consensus criteria)
	ISM-AHN	for SM variants
	SSM-AHN[a]	
	ASM-AHN	
	MCL-AHN	
	According to the AHN:	
	SM with myeloid AHN (SM-CMML, SM-AML,…)	WHO criteria for myeloid AHN type
	SM with lymphoid AHN (SM-ALL, SM-MM,…)	WHO criteria for lymphoid AHN type
ASM	Preceding MC neoplasm (+/−):	≥1 C-finding = ASM
	Primary ASM	No previous SM known
	Secondary ASM	Previous BMM, ISM, SSM, …
	According to an AHN:	
	ASM without AHN	
	ASM-AHN	WHO criteria for AHN
	According to signs of progression:	
	ASM	<5% MC in BM smears
	ASM-T	5%–19% MC in BM smears
MCL	Preceding MC neoplasm (+/−):	≥20% MC in BM or blood smear
	Primary MCL	No previous MC disease known
	Secondary MCL	Previous BMM, ISM, SSM, MCS, …
	According to an AHN:	
	MCL without AHN	
	MCL-AHN	WHO criteria for AHN
	According to organ damage:	
	Chronic MCL	No C-findings
	Acute MCL	One or more C-findings
	According to blood involvement:	MC <10% of blood leukocytes
	Aleukemic MCL	MC ≥ 10% of blood leukocytes
	Leukemic MCL	

Abbreviations: ASM-T, ASM in transformation; CMML, chronic myelomonocytic leukemia; MM, multiple myeloma.

[a] SSM-AHN is an extremely rare condition because signs of myeloproliferation and/or dysplasia will be regarded as sign of the (myeloid) AHN in almost all cases. However, SSM may still be diagnosed in a patient with AHN, for example, when the AHN is a lymphoid neoplasm (eg, SSM-chronic lymphocytic leukemia [CLL]).

Adapted from Valent P, Akin C, Hartmann K, et al. Updated diagnostic criteria and classification of mast cell disorders: a consensus proposal. Hemasphere. 2021;5(11):e646; with permission.

patients, the disease transforms into acute MCL, especially when untreated. Finally, MCL can be divided into pure MCL and MCL-AHN.

It is also important to delineate MCL from true MCS and myelomastocytic leukemia (MML).[95] In patients with MML, SM criteria are not fulfilled; an advanced myeloid neoplasm, such as AML, can be detected; and neoplastic MC are greater than or equal to 10% of all nucleated cells in bone marrow or PB smears.[95] In a subset of patients with MML, *KIT* mutations outside of codon 816 are identified. Some of these

---

Box 2
Diagnostic criteria for mast cell activation syndromes (MCAS)[a]

1. Typical clinical signs of severe, recurrent (episodic) systemic mast cell activation are present, often in the form of anaphylaxis (definition of systemic: involving at least 2 organ systems)

2. Involvement of MC is documented by biochemical studies; preferred marker: increase in serum tryptase level from the individual's baseline to plus 20% (=120%) + 2 ng/mL[b]

3. Response of symptoms to therapy with MC-stabilizing agents, drugs directed against MC mediator production, or drugs blocking mediator release or effects of MC-derived mediators

[a] All 3 MCAS criteria (1+2+3) must be fulfilled to diagnose MCAS. [b] Other MC-derived MC mediators (urinary histamine metabolites, urinary prostaglandin D_2 metabolites) may also serve as markers of systemic mast cell activation. However, these markers are less specific compared with tryptase. *Adapted from* Valent P, Akin C, Hartmann K, et al. Updated diagnostic criteria and classification of mast cell disorders: a consensus proposal. Hemasphere. 2021;5(11):e646; with permission.[37]

---

cases may be reclassified as MCL, because such (KIT-activating) mutations have now been recognized as minor SM criterion.

MCS is a very rare, aggressive localized MC tumor exhibiting a sarcomalike spread with subsequent local organ damage.[31–35,37,97–99] As per definition, no systemic involvement is found and SM criteria are not fulfilled.[31,37] However, despite therapy, most cases progress to MCL within short time.[97–99] Histologically, MCS consists of more or less immature atypical MC that may show signs of proliferation and expand rapidly, often with an invasive (sarcoma-like) infiltration pattern. Any organ system

---

Box 3
Classification of MCAS

Variant of MCAS	Main Diagnostic Features
Primary MCAS (=clonal MCAS= MMAS)[b]	a KIT-activating *KIT* mutation[a] Mast cells express aberrant CD25 (1) with confirmed SM (2) without SM
Secondary MCAS	IgE-dependent allergy or another hypersensitivity disorder or a reactive disease that can trigger mast cell activation
HαT + MCAS (hereditary MCAS)	No underlying disease or condition that could provoke MCAS known and positive HαT test
Mixed forms of MCAS	Combinations of the above-described conditions/ causes demonstrable
Idiopathic MCAS	No contributing factor or condition known/identified

[a] The most prevalent mutation in *KIT* found in these patients is D816V. [b] The terms clonal MCAS and monoclonal MCAS (MMAS) can be usedsynonymously with the term primary MCAS. *Abbreviations:* SM, systemic mastocytosis; HaT, hereditary alpha-tryptasemia.

may be affected. As mentioned, MCS must be delineated distinctively from an MCS-like progression in (advanced) SM. In true MCS, *KIT* mutations are usually absent, whereas *KIT* D816V or other *KIT* mutations are detected in most cases with advanced SM with MCS-like progression.[97–99]

DIAGNOSTIC CRITERIA AND CLASSIFICATION OF MCAS AND RELATED CONDITIONS

Solid diagnostic criteria and a classification for MCAS have been developed between 2010 and 2022 by the consensus group.[12,35,37,62–65] Consensus criteria for MCAS are shown in **Box 2**. These criteria include severe systemic symptoms attributable to MC activation (usually in form of anaphylaxis), an increase in serum tryptase levels to greater than or equal to 120% + 2 ng/mL total over the individual baseline of the patient, and response to drugs targeting MC-derived mediators, MC mediator effects, or MC activation (=MC stabilizer). Based on the underlying cause, genetic background, and known comorbidities, MCAS is divided into primary (monoclonal) MCAS, in which clonal MC are found and SM is usually diagnosed; secondary MCAS, in which an allergic disease or another reactive condition is present; hereditary MCAS, wherein

Table 7
Global classification of mast cell pathologies and related conditions

Disorder/Condition	Diagnostic Criteria/Defining Features
Mast cell hyperplasia	Reactive increase in normal mast cells
	No evidence for clonal mast cells
	Criteria for CM/SM/MCS not fulfilled
Mastocytosis	WHO criteria for CM, SM, or MCS fulfilled
MML	Advanced myeloid neoplasm diagnosed based on WHO criteria (eg, AML) and:
	Increase in neoplastic mast cells ≥10%
	Criteria for CM/SM/MCS not fulfilled
Myelomastocytic expansion in myeloid neoplasms[a]	Myeloid neoplasm diagnosed by WHO criteria[a] and:
	Increase in neoplastic mast cells up to 9% in bone marrow or blood
	Criteria for CM/SM/MCS not fulfilled
MCAS[b]	MCAS criteria fulfilled
	± Criteria for CM/SM/MCS fulfilled
Other MCADs[b]	Evidence for a clinically relevant, local or systemic mast cell activation but the
	criteria for MCAS are not fulfilled[1]
	± Criteria for CM/SM/MCS fulfilled
Predisposing genetic conditions:	
Hereditary alpha tryptasemia (HαT)[c]	Extra gene copy numbers of *TPSAB1*
Hypersensitivity disorders[c]	Allergy with or without specific IgE
Atopic diathesis[c]	Predisposition to develop allergic (hypersensitivity) disorders

[a] In some of these patients, a myeloid/lymphoid neoplasm with a tyrosine kinase gene fusion is found.
[b] MCADs can be divided into MCAS and other MCAD not fulfilling MCAS criteria. The classification of MCAS is shown in **Box 3**.
[c] HαT may predispose to both SM and more severe anaphylaxis (MCAS) in SM contexts, whereas hypersensitivity disorders (allergies) and atopic diathesis only predispose to MCAS but not to SM evolution.
Adapted from Valent P, Akin C, Hartmann K, et al. Updated diagnostic criteria and classification of mast cell disorders: a consensus proposal. Hemasphere. 2021;5(11):e646; with permission.

HαT has been documented; mixed forms of MCAS, wherein multiple underlying causes are detected (eg, SM and an IgE-dependent allergy); and idiopathic MCAS, wherein no known cause can be demonstrated (**Box 3**). The most severe courses, often in the form of recurrent life-threatening anaphylactic events, are found in patients with mixed MCAS. Sometimes, it is difficult to define a final diagnosis.[62–65] More recently, diagnostic algorithms for patients with MCAS and other MC activation disorders have been published.[82,100] Moreover, diagnostic criteria for conditions associated with clinically relevant MC activation not fulfilling (completely) all the diagnostic criteria of MCAS and for conditions predisposing for or mimicking MCAS have been proposed.[82,101] These novel diagnostic tools should assist in daily practice and should facilitate diagnostic work and avoid unnecessary referrals.

GLOBAL CLASSIFICATION OF MAST CELL DISORDERS

In 2012, the consensus group proposed a global classification for all MC disorders for the first time.[62] This classification included not only mastocytosis and MML but also various forms of MCAS.[62] In 2020, the ECNM/AIM consensus group provided an updated version of this global classification.[37] The updated global classification of MC disorders is shown in **Table 7**. In general, MC disorders can be divided into

---

Box 4
Mast cell disorders and predisposing conditions: ICD-10-CM Codes

Disorder/Condition	Abbreviations	ICD-10-CM Code
Mastocytosis:		
Cutaneous mastocytosis	CM	D47.01
Childhood-onset cutaneous mastocytosis	CM	Q82.20
Bone marrow mastocytosis	BMM	D47.02
Indolent systemic mastocytosis	ISM	D47.02
Smoldering systemic mastocytosis	SSM	D47.02
Aggressive systemic mastocytosis	ASM	C96.21
Mast cell leukemia	MCL	C94.30
Mast cell sarcoma	MCS	C96.22
Mastocytoma NOS	-	D47.09
Mast cell activation-related disorders:		
Mast cell activation syndrome	MCAS	D89.40
Mast cell activation, unspecified[a]	MCA-NOS[a]	D89.40[a]
Monoclonal MCAS	MCAS-m	D89.41
Idiopathic MCAS	MCAS-I	D89.42
Secondary/reactive MCAS	MCAS-s/r	D89.43
Other mast cell activation disorders[a]	-	D89.49[a]
New predisposing conditions:		
Hereditary alpha tryptasemia	HαT	D89.44

Abbreviations: ICD, International statistical Classification of Diseases; ICD-10-CM, ICD-10-Clinical Modification; NOS, not otherwise specified.[a]For these conditions, no validated criteria are available to date and the cause of the symptoms usually remains unknown. Therefore, it is important to search for alternative diagnoses and causes in such patients. *Adapted from* Valent P, Akin C, Hartmann K, et al. Updated diagnostic criteria and classification of mast cell disorders: a consensus proposal. Hemasphere. 2021;5(11):e646; with permission.

reactive MC hyperplasia where an increase in nonclonal (reactive) MC can be documented; mastocytosis where an expansion of neoplastic MC is found and diagnostic WHO criteria sufficient to diagnose CM, SM, or a localized form of an MC neoplasm are fulfilled; MML; MCAS; and other MC activation-related disorders (not fulfilling MCAS criteria) (**Table 7**). In addition, an expansion of neoplastic MC in patients with myeloid neoplasms without reaching criteria to diagnose SM or MML may be observed, especially in patients in whom neoplastic cells display a tyrosine kinase fusion, such as *FIP1L1::PDGFRA* (see **Table 7**). Finally, there are MC-related conditions and genetic factors that predispose to the development of SM and/or MCAS, such as HαT, and there are conditions associated with MC activation where MCAS criteria are not fulfilled.[100,101] In their most recent attempt to assist physicians in daily practice and to translate recently updated criteria more rapidly and effectively into practice, the consensus group has made an effort to link their proposed criteria to the International Classification of Diseases-10-Clinical Modification code.[101] The resulting proposed formulation is shown in **Box 4**.

SUMMARY

Mastocytosis is a hematopoietic disease characterized by the expansion and accumulation of neoplastic MC in various organ systems, including the skin, bone marrow, spleen, liver, and GI tract. The diagnostic criteria and classification of mastocytosis proposed by the consensus group (2001–2022) was adopted by the WHO and divides patients into prognostic subsets of CM and SM. Although the basic classification proposed in 2001 remains valid, recent developments in the field and the advent of new diagnostic and prognostic variables and scores have created the need to adjust and refine definitions and criteria in MC neoplasms. Furthermore, MCAS and genetic features predicting the risk of developing SM and MCAS have been described. This article discusses developments and refinements in the criteria and classification of MC disorders proposed by the consensus group that were adopted by the WHO and ICC in 2022.

CLINICS CARE POINTS

- In patients with suspected SM, reliable screening parameters are the basal serum tryptase level and a highly sensitive PCR test for KIT D816V. In those with elevated basal tryptase level and a negative PCR result, genetic testing for HαT is recommended.

- In adult patients with suspected SM and typical skin lesions, a bone marrow investigation is usually recommended. If no bone marrow studies are performed, the provisional diagnosis of MIS can be established.

- When SM is diagnosed, the next step is to establish the variant of SM by applying the diagnostic criteria provided by the consensus group, the WHO, and the ICC.

- In patients with suspected MCAS, consensus MCAS criteria should be applied in each case, and, once diagnosed, the type/variant of MCAS must be established. In those with a clonal MCAS (KIT D816V detectable) an underlying SM is usually present.

AUTHORS' CONTRIBUTIONS

All authors contributed equally by discussing and establishing published articles and the criteria and classification of mast cell disorders. All authors contributed by writing parts of the article, and all authors approved the final version of the document.

CONFLICTS OF INTEREST

In this project: The authors declare that they have no conflicts of interest to disclose. Outside this study: P. Valent: Advisory Board and Honoraria: Novartis, Blueprint Medicines, Deciphera; K. Sotlar: Advisory Board and Honoraria: Novartis, Blueprint Medicines, AstraZeneca; C. Akin: Honoraria: Novartis, Deciphera, Patara; M. Arock: Research Grants: Blueprint Medicines; Advisory Board and Honoraria: AB Science, Blueprint Medicines, ThermoFischer; H.-P. Horny: Advisory Board and Honoraria: Novartis, Deciphera, Blueprint Medicines. The authors declare that they have no other conflicts of interest to disclose.

FUNDING

P. Valent was supported by the Austrian Science Funds, Austria (FWF) grant P32470-B.

ACKNOWLEDGMENTS

The authors thank all European and US experts who joined and actively contributed in the Working Conferences organized by the consensus group in the years 2000, 2005, 2010, 2012, 2015, and 2020. The authors also thank all cooperating scientists and centers in the ECNM and AIM as well as all patient groups and their representatives for their contributions over the past 3 decades.

REFERENCES

1. Metcalfe DD. Mast cells and mastocytosis. Blood 2008;112(4):946–56.
2. Galli SJ, Tsai M. Mast cells in allergy and infection: versatile effector and regulatory cells in innate and adaptive immunity. Eur J Immunol 2010;40(7):1843–51.
3. Theoharides TC, Valent P, Akin C. Mast cells, mastocytosis, and related disorders. N Engl J Med 2015;373(2):163–72.
4. Valent P, Akin C, Hartmann K, et al. Mast cells as a unique hematopoietic lineage and cell system: From Paul Ehrlich's visions to precision medicine concepts. Theranostics 2020;10(23):10743–68.
5. Galli SJ, Gaudenzio N, Tsai M. Mast cells in inflammation and disease: recent progress and ongoing concerns. Annu Rev Immunol 2020;38:49–77.
6. Valent P, Bettelheim P. Cell surface structures on human basophils and mast cells: biochemical and functional characterization. Adv Immunol 1992;52: 333–423.
7. Galli SJ. New concepts about the mast cell. N Engl J Med 1993;328(4):257–65.
8. Horny HP, Sotlar K, Valent P. Mastocytosis: state of the art. Pathobiology 2007; 74(2):121–32.
9. Arock M, Valent P. Pathogenesis, classification and treatment of mastocytosis: state of the art in 2010 and future perspectives. Expert Rev Hematol 2010; 3(4):497–516.
10. Akin C, Valent P. Diagnostic criteria and classification of mastocytosis in 2014. Immunol Allergy Clin North Am 2014;34(2):207–18.
11. Hartmann K, Escribano L, Grattan C, et al. Cutaneous manifestations in patients with mastocytosis: Consensus report of the European Competence Network on Mastocytosis; the American Academy of Allergy, Asthma & Immunology; and the European Academy of Allergology and Clinical Immunology. J Allergy Clin Immunol 2016;137(1):35–45.

12. Valent P, Akin C, Hartmann K, et al. Advances in the classification and treatment of mastocytosis: current status and outlook toward the future. Cancer Res 2017; 77(6):1261–70.

13. Nettleship E, Tay W. Rare forms of urticaria. Br Med J 1869;2:323–4.

14. Ehrlich P. Beiträge zur Kenntnis der granulierten Bindegewebszellen und der eosinophilen Leukocyten. Arch Anat Physiol 1879;7:166–9.

15. Unna PG. Beitrage zur Anatomie und Pathogeneses der Urticaria Simplex und Pigmentosa. Monatschr Prakt Dermatol Suppl Dermatol 1887;3:9.

16. Ellis JM. Urticaria pigmentosa; a report of a case with autopsy. ArchPathol 1949; 48:426–35.

17. Valent P, Akin C, Sperr WR, et al. Smouldering mastocytosis: a novel subtype of systemic mastocytosis with slow progression. Int Arch Allergy Immunol 2002; 127(2):137–9.

18. Sotlar K, Colak S, Bache A, et al. Variable presence of KITD816V in clonal hae-matological non-mast cell lineage diseases associated with systemic mastocy-tosis (SM-AHNMD). J Pathol 2010;220(5):586–95.

19. Georgin-Lavialle S, Lhermitte L, Dubreuil P, et al. Mast cell leukemia. Blood 2013;121(8):1285–95.

20. Monnier J, Georgin-Lavialle S, Canioni D, et al. Mast cell sarcoma: new cases and literature review. Oncotarget 2016;7(40):66299–309.

21. Schwartz LB, Irani AM. Serum tryptase and the laboratory diagnosis of systemic mastocytosis. Hematol Oncol Clin North Am 2000;14(3):641–57.

22. Nagata H, Worobec AS, Oh CK, et al. Identification of a point mutation in the cat-alytic domain of the protooncogene c-kit in peripheral blood mononuclear cells of patients who have mastocytosis with an associated hematologic disorder. Proc Natl Acad Sci (USA) 1995;92(23):10560–4.

23. Longley BJ, Tyrrell L, Lu SZ, et al. Somatic c-KIT activating mutation in urticaria pigmentosa and aggressive mastocytosis: establishment of clonality in a human mast cell neoplasm. Nat Genet 1996;12(3):312–4.

24. Sotlar K, Marafioti T, Griesser H, et al. Detection of c-kit mutation Asp 816 to Val in microdissected bone marrow infiltrates in a case of systemic mastocytosis associated with chronic myelomonocytic leukaemia. Mol Pathol 2000;53(4): 188–93.

25. Fritsche-Polanz R, Jordan JH, Feix A, et al. Mutation analysis of C-KIT in patients with myelodysplastic syndromes without mastocytosis and cases of systemic mastocytosis. Br J Haematol 2001;113(2):357–64.

26. Horny HP, Sillaber C, Menke D, et al. Diagnostic value of immunostaining for tryptase in patients with mastocytosis. Am J Surg Pathol 1998;22(9):1132–40.

27. Escribano L, Orfao A, Díaz-Agustin B, et al. Indolent systemic mast cell disease in adults: immunophenotypic characterization of bone marrow mast cells and its diagnostic implications. Blood 1998;91(8):2731–6.

28. Sperr WR, Escribano L, Jordan JH, et al. Morphologic properties of neoplastic mast cells: delineation of stages of maturation and implication for cytological grading of mastocytosis. Leuk Res 2001;25(7):529–36.

29. Sperr WR, Jordan JH, Fiegl M, et al. Serum tryptase levels in patients with mas-tocytosis: correlation with mast cell burden and implication for defining the cate-gory of disease. Int Arch Allergy Immunol 2002;128:136–41.

30. Valent P, Escribano L, Parwaresch RM, et al. Recent advances in mastocytosis research. Summary of the Vienna Mastocytosis Meeting 1998. Int Arch Allergy Immunol 1999;120:1–7.

31. Valent P, Horny HP, Escribano L, et al. Diagnostic criteria and classification of mastocytosis: a consensus proposal. Leuk Res 2001;25:603–25.
32. Valent P, Horny H-P, Li CY, et al. Mastocytosis (mast cell disease). In: Jaffe ES, Harris NL, Stein H, et al, editors. World Health Organization (WHO) classification of Tumours. Pathology & genetics. Tumours of Haematopoietic and lymphoid tissues. Lyon (France): IARC Press; 2001. p. 291–302.
33. Horny HP, Akin C, Metcalfe DD, et al. Mastocytosis (mast cell disease). In: Swerdlow SH, Campo E, Harris NL, et al, editors. World Health Organization (WHO) classification of Tumours. Pathology & genetics. Tumours of Haematopoietic and lymphoid tissues. Lyon (France): IARC Press; 2008. p. 54–63.
34. Horny HP, Akin C, Arber D, et al. Mastocytosis. In: Swerdlow SH, Campo E, Harris NL, et al, editors. WHO classification of Tumours of Haematopoietic and lymphoid tissues. Lyon (France): IARC Press; 2017. p. 62–9.
35. Valent P, Akin C, Metcalfe DD, et al. 2016 updated WHO classification and novel emerging treatment concepts. Blood 2017;129:1420–7.
36. Reiter A, George TI, Gotlib J. New developments in diagnosis, prognostication, and treatment of advanced systemic mastocytosis. Blood 2020;135:1365–76.
37. Valent P, Akin C, Hartmann K, et al. Updated diagnostic criteria and classification of mast cell disorders: a consensus proposal. Hemasphere 2021;5(11): e646.
38. Khoury JD, Solary E, Abla O, et al. The 5th edition of the World Health Organization Classification of Haematolymphoid Tumours: Myeloid and Histiocytic/Dendritic Neoplasms. Leukemia 2022;36(7):1703–19.
39. Wilson TM, Maric I, Simakova O, et al. Clonal analysis of NRAS activating mutations in KIT-D816V systemic mastocytosis. Haematologica 2011;96:459–63.
40. Traina F, Visconte V, Jankowska AM, et al. Single nucleotide polymorphism array lesions, TET2, DNMT3A, ASXL1 and CBL mutations are present in systemic mastocytosis. PLoS One 2012;7:e43090.
41. Schwaab J, Schnittger S, Sotlar K, et al. Comprehensive mutational profiling in advanced systemic mastocytosis. Blood 2013;122:2460–6.
42. Damaj G, Joris M, Chandesris O, et al. ASXL1 but not TET2 mutations adversely impact overall survival of patients suffering systemic mastocytosis with associated clonal hematologic non-mast-cell diseases. PLoS One 2014;9:e85362.
43. Jawhar M, Schwaab J, Schnittger S, et al. Additional mutations in SRSF2, ASXL1 and/or RUNX1 identify a high-risk group of patients with KIT D816V(+) advanced systemic mastocytosis. Leukemia 2016;30:136–43.
44. Jawhar M, Döhner K, Kreil S, et al. KIT D816 mutated/CBF-negative acute myeloid leukemia: a poor-risk subtype associated with systemic mastocytosis. Leukemia 2019;33:1124–34.
45. Naumann N, Jawhar M, Schwaab J, et al. Incidence and prognostic impact of cytogenetic aberrations in patients with systemic mastocytosis. Genes Chromosomes Cancer 2018;57:252–9.
46. Pardanani A, Lasho T, Elala Y, et al. Next-generation sequencing in systemic mastocytosis: Derivation of a mutation-augmented clinical prognostic model for survival. Am J Hematol 2016;91:888–93.
47. Muñoz-González JI, Álvarez-Twose I, Jara-Acevedo M, et al. Frequency and prognostic impact of KIT and other genetic variants in indolent systemic mastocytosis. Blood 2019;134:456–68.
48. Kluin-Nelemans HC, Jawhar M, Reiter A, et al. Cytogenetic and molecular aberrations and worse outcome for male patients in systemic mastocytosis. Theranostics 2021;11:292–303.

49. Sperr WR, Kundi M, Alvarez-Twose I, et al. International prognostic scoring system for mastocytosis (IPSM): a retrospective cohort study. Lancet Haematol 2019;6:e638–49.

50. Jawhar M, Schwaab J, Álvarez-Twose I, et al. MARS: Mutation-Adjusted Risk Score for Advanced Systemic Mastocytosis. J Clin Oncol 2019;37:2846–56.

51. Muñoz-González JI, Álvarez-Twose I, Jara-Acevedo M, et al. Proposed global prognostic score for systemic mastocytosis: a retrospective prognostic modelling study. Lancet Haematol 2021;8:e194–204.

52. Bonadonna P, Gonzalez-de-Olano D, Zanotti R, et al. Venom immunotherapy in patients with clonal mast cell disorders: efficacy, safety, and practical considerations. J Allergy Clin Immunol Pract 2013;1:474–8.

53. Ustun C, Reiter A, Scott BL, et al. Hematopoietic stem-cell transplantation for advanced systemic mastocytosis. J Clin Oncol 2014;32:3264–74.

54. Alvarez-Twose I, Martínez-Barranco P, Gotlib J, et al. Complete response to gemtuzumab ozogamicin in a patient with refractory mast cell leukemia. Leukemia 2016;30:1753–6.

55. Gotlib J, Kluin-Nelemans HC, George TI, et al. Efficacy and Safety of Midostaurin in Advanced Systemic Mastocytosis. N Engl J Med 2016;374:2530–41.

56. Valent P, Akin C, Hartmann K, et al. Midostaurin: a magic bullet that blocks mast cell expansion and activation. Ann Oncol 2017;28:2367–76.

57. Jendoubi F, Gaudenzio N, Gallini A, et al. Omalizumab in the treatment of adult patients with mastocytosis: A systematic review. Clin Exp Allergy 2020;50: 654–61.

58. Gotlib J, Reiter A, Radia DH, et al. Efficacy and safety of avapritinib in advanced systemic mastocytosis: interim analysis of the phase 2 PATHFINDER trial. Nat Med 2021;27(12):2192–9.

59. Reiter A, Schwaab J, DeAngelo DJ, et al. Efficacy and safety of avapritinib in previously treated patients with advanced systemic mastocytosis. Blood Adv 2022;6(21):5750–62.

60. Reiter A, Gotlib J, Álvarez-Twose I, et al. Efficacy of avapritinib versus best available therapy in the treatment of advanced systemic mastocytosis. Leukemia 2022;36(8):2108–20.

61. Gotlib J, Reiter A, DeAngelo DJ. Avapritinib for advanced systemic mastocytosis. Blood 2022;140(15):1667–73.

62. Valent P, Akin C, Arock M, et al. Definitions, criteria and global classification of mast cell disorders with special reference to mast cell activation syndromes: a consensus proposal. Int Arch Allergy Immunol 2012;157:215–25.

63. Akin C, Valent P, Metcalfe DD. Mast cell activation syndrome: Proposed diagnostic criteria. J Allergy Clin Immunol 2010;126:1099–104.e4.

64. Valent P. Mast cell activation syndromes: definition and classification. Allergy 2013;68:417–24.

65. Valent P, Akin C, Nedoszytko B, et al. Diagnosis, classification and management of mast cell activation syndromes (MCAS) in the era of personalized medicine. Int J Mol Sci 2020;21:9030.

66. Lyons JJ, Yu X, Hughes JD, et al. Elevated basal serum tryptase identifies a multisystem disorder associated with increased TPSAB1 copy number. Nat Genet 2016;48:1564–9.

67. Lyons JJ. Hereditary Alpha Tryptasemia: Genotyping and Associated Clinical Features. Immunol Allergy Clin North Am 2018;38:483–95.

68. Lyons JJ, Chovanec J, O'Connell MP, et al. Heritable risk for severe anaphylaxis associated with increased alpha-tryptase-encoding germline copy number at TPSAB1. J Allergy Clin Immunol 2021;147:622–32.

69. Greiner G, Sprinzl B, Górska A, et al. Hereditary α tryptasemia is a valid genetic biomarker for severe mediator-related symptoms in mastocytosis. Blood 2021; 137:238–47.

70. Bonadonna P, Perbellini O, Passalacqua G, et al. Clonal mast cell disorders in patients with systemic reactions to Hymenoptera stings and increased serum tryptase levels. J Allergy Clin Immunol 2009;123:680–6.

71. Bonadonna P, Zanotti R, Müller U. Mastocytosis and insect venom allergy. Curr Opin Allergy Clin Immunol 2010;10:347–53.

72. Wimazal F, Geissler P, Shnawa P, et al. Severe life-threatening or disabling anaphylaxis in patients with systemic mastocytosis: a single-center experience. Int Arch Allergy Immunol 2012;157:399–405.

73. Alvarez-Twose I, Bonadonna P, Matito A, et al. Systemic mastocytosis as a risk factor for severe hymenoptera sting-induced anaphylaxis. J Allergy Clin Immunol 2013;131:614–5.

74. Zanotti R, Lombardo C, Passalacqua G, et al. Clonal mast cell disorders in patients with severe Hymenoptera venom allergy and normal serum tryptase levels. J Allergy Clin Immunol 2015;136:135–9.

75. Valent P, Akin C, Escribano L, et al. Standards and standardization in mastocytosis: consensus statements on diagnostics, treatment recommendations and response criteria. Eur J Clin Invest 2007;37:435–53.

76. Akin C, Fumo G, Yavuz AS, et al. A novel form of mastocytosis associated with a transmembrane c-kit mutation and response to imatinib. Blood 2004;103: 3222–5.

77. Álvarez-Twose I, Jara-Acevedo M, Morgado JM, et al. Clinical, immunophenotypic, and molecular characteristics of well-differentiated systemic mastocytosis. J Allergy Clin Immunol 2016;137:168–78.e1.

78. Alvarez-Twose I, Matito A, Morgado JM, et al. Imatinib in systemic mastocytosis: a phase IV clinical trial in patients lacking exon 17 KIT mutations and review of the literature. Oncotarget 2016;8:68950–63.

79. Huang L, Wang SA, Konoplev S, et al. Well-differentiated systemic mastocytosis showed excellent clinical response to imatinib in the absence of known molecular genetic abnormalities: a case report. Medicine (Baltim) 2016;95:e4934.

80. Arber DA, Orazi A, Hasserjian RP, et al. International Consensus Classification of myeloid neoplasms and acute leukemias: integrating morphologic, clinical, and genomic data. Blood 2022;140(11):1200–28.

81. Valent P, Escribano L, Broesby-Olsen S, et al. Proposed diagnostic algorithm for patients with suspected mastocytosis: a proposal of the European Competence Network on Mastocytosis. Allergy 2014;69:1267–74.

82. Valent P, Hartmann K, Schwaab J, et al. Personalized management strategies in mast cell disorders: ECNM-AIM user's guide for daily clinical practice. J Allergy Clin Immunol Pract 2022;10(8):1999–2012.e6.

83. Aberer E, Sperr WR, Bretterklieber A, et al. Clinical Impact of Skin Lesions in Mastocytosis: A Multicenter Study of the European Competence Network on Mastocytosis. Invest Dermatol 2021;141(7):1719–27.

84. Wiechers T, Rabenhorst A, Schick T, et al. Large maculopapular cutaneous lesions are associated with favorable outcome in childhood-onset mastocytosis. J Allergy Clin Immunol 2015;136:1581–90.

85. Sotlar K, Cerny-Reiterer S, Petat-Dutter K, et al. Aberrant expression of CD30 in neoplastic mast cells in high-grade mastocytosis. Mod Pathol 2011;24:585–95.
86. Valent P, Sotlar K, Horny HP. Aberrant expression of CD30 in aggressive systemic mastocytosis and mast cell leukemia: a differential diagnosis to consider in aggressive hematopoietic CD30-positive neoplasms. Leuk Lymphoma 2011; 52:740–4.
87. Morgado JM, Perbellini O, Johnson RC, et al. CD30 expression by bone marrow mast cells from different diagnostic variants of systemic mastocytosis. Histopathology 2013;63:780–7.
88. Blatt K, Cerny-Reiterer S, Schwaab J, et al. Identification of the Ki-1 antigen (CD30) as a novel therapeutic target in systemic mastocytosis. Blood 2015; 126:2832–41.
89. Arock M, Sotlar K, Akin C, et al. KIT mutation analysis in mast cell neoplasms: recommendations of the European Competence Network on Mastocytosis. Leukemia 2015;29:1223–32.
90. Garcia-Montero AC, Jara-Acevedo M, Teodosio C, et al. KIT mutation in mast cells and other bone marrow hematopoietic cell lineages in systemic mast cell disorders: a prospective study of the Spanish Network on Mastocytosis (REMA) in a series of 113 patients. Blood 2006;108:2366–72.
91. Bodemer C, Hermine O, Palmérini F, et al. Pediatric mastocytosis is a clonal disease associated with D816V and other activating c-KIT mutations. J Invest Dermatol 2010;130:804–15.
92. Arock M, Hoermann G, Sotlar K, et al. Clinical impact and proposed application of molecular markers, genetic variants, and cytogenetic analysis in mast cell neoplasms: status 2022. J Allergy Clin Immunol 2022;149:1855–65.
93. Zanotti R, Bonifacio M, Lucchini G, et al. Refined diagnostic criteria for bone marrow mastocytosis: a proposal of the European competence network on mastocytosis. Leukemia 2022;36:516–24.
94. Trizuljak J, Sperr WR, Nekvindová L, et al. Clinical features and survival of patients with indolent systemic mastocytosis defined by the updated WHO classification. Allergy 2020;75:1927–38.
95. Valent P, Sotlar K, Sperr WR, et al. Refined diagnostic criteria and classification of mast cell leukemia (MCL) and myelomastocytic leukemia (MML): a consensus proposal. Ann Oncol 2014;25:1691–700.
96. Sperr WR, Horny HP, Valent P. Spectrum of associated clonal hematologic non-mast cell lineage disorders occurring in patients with systemic mastocytosis. Int Arch Allergy Immunol 2002;127:140–2.
97. Horny HP, Parwaresch MR, Kaiserling E, et al. Mast cell sarcoma of the larynx. J Clin Pathol 1986;39:596–602.
98. Chott A, Guenther P, Huebner A, et al. Morphologic and immunophenotypic properties of neoplastic cells in a case of mast cell sarcoma. Am J Surg Pathol 2003;27:1013–9.
99. Georgin-Lavialle S, Aguilar C, Guieze R, et al. Mast cell sarcoma: a rare and aggressive entity–report of two cases and review of the literature. J Clin Oncol 2013;31:e90–7.
100. Valent P, Akin C, Bonadonna P, et al. Proposed diagnostic algorithm for patients with suspected mast cell activation syndrome. J Allergy Clin Immunol Pract 2019;7:1125–11233.e1.
101. Valent P, Hartmann K, Bonadonna P, et al. Global classification of mast cell activation disorders: an ICD-10-CM-adjusted proposal of the ECNM-AIM consortium. J Allergy Clin Immunol Pract 2022;10:1941–50.

KIT Mutations and Other Genetic Defects in Mastocytosis

Implications for Disease Pathology and Targeted Therapies

Yannick Chantran, PharmD, PhD[a,b,c], Peter Valent, MD[d,e],
Michel Arock, PharmD, PhD[a,f,*]

KEYWORDS

- Mast cells • Mastocytosis • *KIT* D816V mutation • Mutation burden • ASO-qPCR
- ddPCR • Tyrosine kinase inhibitors

KEY POINTS

- Mastocytosis is a group of rare diseases characterized by abnormal accumulation/proliferation of mast cells (MC) in one or several organs.
- In adults, mastocytosis is mostly systemic (systemic mastocytosis; SM) and chronic, affecting the bone marrow (BM) and other internal organs, with or without skin involvement.
- Acquired *KIT* mutations (mostly *KIT* D816V) are the unique genetic defect found in the vast majority of indolent SM, whereas additional myeloid malignancy-related genetic defect(s) are frequently found in advanced forms of the disease (advanced variants of SM [AdvSM]).

Continued

INTRODUCTION

Mastocytosis is a group of rare diseases characterized by abnormal expansion of neoplastic mast cells (MC) in at least one organ/tissue, mainly skin, bone marrow (BM), and gastrointestinal tract.[1] Mastocytosis can affect both children and adults.

[a] Department of Biological Hematology, Pitié-Salpêtrière Hospital, DMU BioGem, AP-HP.Sorbonne University, Paris, France; [b] Department of Biological Immunology, Saint-Antoine Hospital, DMU BioGem, AP-HP.Sorbonne University, Paris, France; [c] Health Environmental Risk Assessment (HERA) Team, Centre of Research in Epidemiology and Statistics (CRESS), Inserm / INRAE, Faculty of Pharmacy, Université de Paris, Paris, France; [d] Ludwig Boltzmann Institute for Hematology and Oncology, Medical University of Vienna, Austria; [e] Division of Hematology and Hemostaseology, Department of Internal Medicine, Medical University of Vienna; [f] Department of Biological Hematology, Pitié-Salpêtrière Hospital, DMU BioGem, AP-HP.Sorbonne University, Paris, France
* Corresponding author. Department of Biological Hematology, DMU BioGem, Pitié-Salpêtrière Charles-Foix Hospital, AP-HP.Sorbonne University, 47/83 Bd de l'Hôpital, Paris 75013.
E-mail address: michel.arock@aphp.fr

Immunol Allergy Clin N Am 43 (2023) 651–664
https://doi.org/10.1016/j.iac.2023.04.008
0889-8561/23/© 2023 Elsevier Inc. All rights reserved.

Continued

- Highly sensitive and quantitative techniques such as allele specific-quantitative PCR or droplet digital PCR are recommended to detect and quantify the *KIT* D816V mutant in various tissues, including peripheral blood (PB) and BM, allowing diagnosis, prognostication, and follow-up of patients with SM.
- In SM, including AdvSM, patients may benefit from treatment with KIT-targeting tyrosine kinase inhibitors, and the treatment efficacy may be assessed by monitoring *KIT* D816V mutational burden in PB and/or BM.

Most pediatric and adult patients display *KIT* activating mutations in neoplastic MC.[2] The *KIT* D816V mutation is the most frequently detected (>80% of the cases) in systemic mastocytosis (SM), a category of mastocytosis mainly found in adult patients.[2] This mutant can be detected in BM, peripheral blood (PB) and infiltrated tissues with highly sensitive and quantitative techniques, that is, allele specific quantitative-(RT) PCR (ASO-qRT-PCR on mRNA or allele specific-quantitative PCR [ASO-qPCR] on DNA),[3,4] or droplet digital PCR (ddPCR) on DNA.[5] These techniques contribute to diagnosis, prognosis, and follow-up of patients and are thus considered as reference techniques.[6] Although the *KIT* D816V mutant is usually the unique genetic defect found in indolent variant of SM (indolent SM [ISM]), patients with more advanced variants of SM (AdvSM) have often additional genetic defects in other myeloid malignancy-related genes apart *KIT*.[7] These defects, usually associated with worse prognosis,[7] are best evidenced by next-generation sequencing (NGS).[8]

Of note, 2 KIT-targeted tyrosine kinase inhibitors (KIT-TKIs), namely midostaurin (Rydapt),[9] and avapritinib (Ayvakit),[10] are now approved by FDA and European Medlines Agency (EMA) to treat AdvSM. In the era of such KIT-TKIs, the monitoring of the *KIT* D816V mutational burden has become one of the most potent markers to evaluate treatment response.

In this review, after a brief overview of the diagnosis and classification of mastocytosis, we will summarize the role of *KIT* and non-*KIT* mutations in the physiopathology of SM. We will then describe the methods currently available not only to detect the *KIT* D816V mutation but also to quantify the mutation burden and to monitor the treatment of AdvSM patients with KIT-TKIs. As a conclusion and perspective part, we will point to the question of the definition of molecular responses (MRs) in patients treated with these drugs.

DIAGNOSTIC CRITERIA AND CLASSIFICATION OF MASTOCYTOSIS

Please refer to the article by Valent and colleagues, "WHO Classification and Diagnosis of Mastocytosis: Update 2023 and Future Perspectives," in this issue for a detailed background of the most updated classification and diagnostic criteria for mastocytosis. Briefly, mastocytosis is classified into 3 major categories: cutaneous mastocytosis (CM), SM, and a very rare category of localized MC neoplasms, namely MC sarcoma (MCS), a very aggressive localized neoplasm composed of highly atypical MC.[11] The diagnosis of CM in pediatric patients requires the presence of typical skin lesions, positive Darier's sign, the absence of systemic involvement and, unlike in adults, rarely requires skin or BM biopsy.[12,13] Conversely, in adults, mastocytosis in skin is mostly found as part of SM.[14]

Historical criteria for the diagnosis of SM[15] have been amended recently.[16] Variants of SM are defined according to (1) the presence or absence of high disease burden

(B-findings) and organ involvement (C-findings), (2) the presence or absence of an associated hematologic neoplasm (AHN), and (3) percentage of MC in BM or PB smears.[16–18] Of note, aggressive SM (ASM), mast cell leukemia (MCL), and SM with an associated hematologic neoplasm (SM-AHN) are collectively termed advanced SM (AdvSM).[19] Besides, well-differentiated SM (WDSM), a morphologic variant characterized by compact multifocal infiltrates of round mature MC in BM and constant skin involvement, may occur in any SM type/subtype.[20]

THE ROLE OF *KIT* MUTATIONS IN THE PATHOPHYSIOLOGY OF MASTOCYTOSIS

In human, the *KIT* gene is located on the long arm of chromosome 4 (4q11–4q13) and contains 21 exons that span overall 80 kb of DNA (**Fig. 1**).[21] *KIT* encodes a 976 amino acid transmembrane tyrosine kinase receptor, capable of activating mitogenic signals when stimulated by its ligand, the stem cell factor (SCF).[22] KIT plays a critical role in

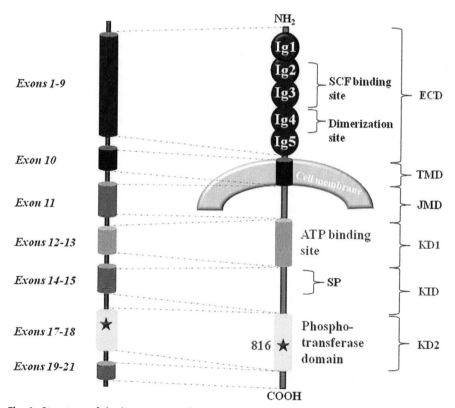

Fig. 1. Structure of the human normal *KIT* gene and of the corresponding KIT receptor. The *KIT* gene (left) contains 21 exons and encodes for KIT, the stem cell factor (SCF) receptor (right). The extracellular domain (ECD; in violet) display 5 immunoglobulin (Ig)-like subunits including a ligand binding site for SCF, and a dimerization site. After a TMD (in brown) made by a single helix, the cytoplasmic region contains an auto-inhibitory juxta-membrane domain (JMD), and a kinase domain (KD) split by a large kinase insert domain (KID) into KD1 (ATP-binding site in gray), and KD2 (phosphotransferase domain in yellow; PTD). The "Switch Pocket" (SP) allows the kinase to adopt an active or inactive conformation. The position of the most common *KIT* mutation (D816V) found in >80% of all patients with SM is highlighted by a red star.

the development of MC, melanocytes, hematopoietic stem cells, germ cells, and interstitial cells of Cajal.[23–26] In hematopoietic processes, KIT is involved in the differentiation of myeloid and lymphoid cells from hematopoietic stem cells and is downregulated on mature cells, excepted for MC.[27] The KIT receptor is composed of an extracellular domain (ECD) characterized by 5 Ig-like domains containing a ligand-binding site for SCF and a dimerization site (see **Fig. 1**). The ECD is linked to a cytoplasmic region by a short transmembrane domain (TMD; see **Fig. 1**). The cytoplasmic region consists of a juxtamembrane domain (JMD) and a bipartite tyrosine kinase domain where the ATP binding site and the phosphotransferase domain (PTD) are separated by a kinase-insert (see **Fig. 1**).[21] SCF binding to KIT leads to dimerization and autophosphorylation of the receptor at tyrosine residues serving as docking sites for signal transduction molecules.[28] The transduction process involves multiple signaling pathways such as PI3-kinase, Src family kinase, Ras-Erk, and JAK/STAT, resulting in cell proliferation, survival, and migration.[28]

KIT D816V and Other KIT Mutations in Mastocytosis

More than 80% of all patients with SM harbor the KIT D816V mutation.[29] In ISM and smoldering SM (SSM), this mutation is retrieved in virtually all the patients and is usually the only genetic anomaly detected in neoplastic MC.[29] Other variants at codon 816 have been found occasionally in ISM/SSM.[29] In AdvSM, although the KIT D816V mutant is found in greater than 80% of the patients, additional mutations at other KIT codons or no KIT mutations have been reported, particularly in MCL cases. Indeed, in a recent study, among 85 patients with MCL evaluated for KIT structure, KIT D816V was found in 73% of the patients, 11% of the individuals had alternative KIT mutations, and 17% were KIT wild type.[30] In addition, in most patients with WDSM, no KIT mutations are found, whereas KIT D816V or other KIT mutants may be detected in only ~30% of the patients.[20]

In contrast to adult SM, the KIT D816V mutant is found in ~30% of children in skin biopsies.[31] Other KIT mutations, mainly located in the ECD of the receptor, are found in ~40% of all cases with childhood CM or SM.[31,32] Thus, ~70% of childhood patients with mastocytosis have KIT defects, confirming that pediatric mastocytosis is also a clonal disease similar to SM in adults but with a broader spectrum of KIT mutations.[12]

Finally, regarding MCS, in the largest cohort reported to date, KIT mutational status was investigated in 14 patients and showed the absence of mutations in 50% of the cases, KIT D816V mutation in 21% of the patients and non-816 mutants in the remaining cases.[33]

A comparison of the frequency and nature of the various KIT defects found in pediatric versus adult patients with mastocytosis is presented in **Fig. 2**.

Impact of the KIT D816V Mutant Receptor on Cell Survival and Proliferation

It is far beyond the scope of this review to detail the signaling pathways aberrantly recruited by the KIT D816V mutant receptor. Briefly, the D816V gain of function mutation leads to a conformational change in the PTD, which entails constitutive activation of the receptor, independently of its dimerization.[34] Key downstream signaling pathways aberrantly activated by oncogenic KIT D816V mutant comprise, among others, PI3-kinase/protein kinase B (AKT),[35] signal transducer and activator of transcription-5 (STAT-5),[36] nuclear factor-kappa B (NF-kB),[37] mammalian target of rapamycin complex 2,[38] and rotein kinase C-delta (PKCδ).[39] In addition, the abnormal accumulation of neoplastic MC in SM could result from the deregulation of proapoptotic and antiapoptotic pathways. There is evidence of overexpression of the antiapoptotic

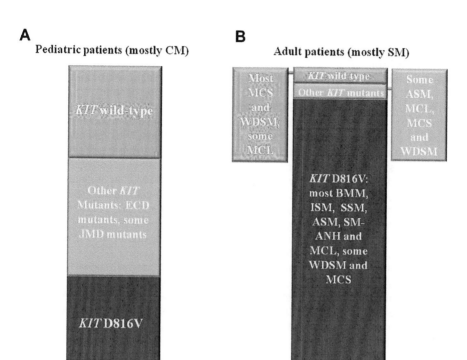

Fig. 2. Differential repartition of *KIT* mutations between pediatric and adult patients and, in adults, between SM variants. In pediatric patients (panel *A*), the *KIT* D816V mutant is found in ~30% of the cases, whereas ~40% of the patients harbor non-*KIT* D816V mutants, principally located in the ECD of KIT. Finally, 30% of the pediatric patients are *KIT* wild-type. By contrast, in adults (panel *B*), greater than 80% of all patients with SM harbor the *KIT* D816V mutation, as found in BM and/or PB, whereas patients with MCL, MCS, and moreover in the WDSM variant harbor slightly less frequently the *KIT* D816V mutation. ASM, aggressive SM; BM, bone marrow; BMM, bone marrow mastocytosis; ISM, indolent SM; MCL, mast cell leukemia; MCS, mast cell sarcoma; PB, peripheral blood; SM, systemic mastocytosis; SM-AHN, SM with an associated hematologic neoplasm; SSM, smouldering SM; WDSM, well-differentiated SM; WT, wild type.

molecules B-cell leukemia/lymphoma 2 (BCL-2), BCL-xL, and MCL-1 in *KIT* D816V-positive neoplastic MC in SM patients.[40,41] In contrast, a loss of expression of the pro-apoptotic Bcl-2 interacting mediator of cell death (BIM) molecule is detected in these cells.[42] All these signaling and antiapoptotic pathways aberrantly evoked by the KIT D81V mutant receptor may concur to the abnormal accumulation/proliferation/survival of neoplastic MC in mastocytosis.[43]

THE ROLE OF NON-*KIT* MUTATIONS IN THE PATHOPHYSIOLOGY AND PROGNOSIS OF DIFFERENT SYSTEMIC MASTOCYTOSIS VARIANTS

Nearly 90% of patients with AdvSM and *KIT* D816V have additional somatic mutations (eg, *JAK2* V617F, *FIPL1-PDGFRA*, *BCR-ABL1*, *TET2*, *SRSF2*, *ASXL1*, *EZH2*, *CBL*, *RUNX1*, *RAS*), most with an SM-AHN.[7] In contrast, these additional mutations are rarely seen in patients with SSM or ISM.[44,45] They can be divided into lesions in disease-specific driver genes such as *JAK2* V617F, *FIPL1-PDGFRA*, or *BCR-ABL1* and lesions in genes not specific for a distinct hematological myeloid neoplasm.

Lesions in disease-related driver genes are found almost exclusively in SM-AHN where they define the nature and variant of the AHN.[46–49] However, other molecular aberrations repeatedly reported in patients with AdvSM, mostly in SM-AHN and to a lesser extent in ASM and MCL,[7,50–55] may affect signaling molecules (eg, *CBL*, *KRAS*, or *NRAS*), transcription factors (eg, *RUNX1*), epigenetic regulators (eg, *ASXL1*, *DNMT3A*, *EZH2*, or *TET2*), splicing factors (eg, *SRSF2*, *SF3B1*, or *U2AF1*) (reviewed in ref.[56]) or the tumor suppressor *SETD2*.[57] Several groups have investigated the prognostic relevance of these additional mutations. The presence and number of mutated genes within the *SRSF2/ASXL1/RUNX1* (S/A/R) panel,[58] the presence of mutations in *ASXL1* and/or *CBL*,[55] and *EZH2* gene mutations in addition to the S/A/R genes panel are associated with inferior survival in AdvSM.[59] In addition, although rarely found, mutations in the S/A/R genes panel together with mutations in *DNMT3A* are associated with poor outcome in patients with ISM and SSM.[45,59] Thus, nowadays, there is a consensus opinion that not only patients with AdvSM but also those with bone marrow mastocytosis (BMM), ISM, and SSM should have a myeloid NGS panel investigation, preferably from BM.[6]

Of note, highlighting the deleterious nature of some of these additional genetic defects has led to their incorporation into new mixed clinical, biochemical, and molecular prognostic scoring systems, such as the Mayo Alliance Prognostic System,[60] the Red Española de Mastocitosis (REMA) score,[59] the Mutation-Adjusted Risk Score,[58] or the Global Prognostic score for SM.[45]

METHODS TO DETECT (AND QUANTIFY) *KIT* MUTATIONS IN MASTOCYTOSIS

The *KIT* D816V mutant being by far the most frequent *KIT* defect retrieved in the major categories of SM, highly sensitive techniques targeting the detection of this particular mutant are recommended in first line.[6,61] Diagnostic standard is mutation analysis of *KIT* on BM aspirate, and if not available, on BM smear or formalin-fixed paraffin-embedded (FFPE) biopsy sample.[62] However, with the recently developed ASO-qPCR/ddPCR sensitive techniques, the *KIT* D816V mutant can also be detected in PB in most patients with SM, making PB testing the first-line test to be carried out in case of suspicion of SM.[6] Pros and cons of different methods able to detect the D816V mutation in at least 80% of patients with SM; therefore, candidates to be used for routine testing are summarized in **Table 1**.[63–66]

The most sensitive methods for the identification and quantization (mutational burden) of the *KIT* D816V mutation in different samples, including BM samples, PB and FFPE tissues, are ASO-qPCR and ddPCR. They allow detecting less than 0.01% *KIT* D816V mutation-positive cells.[3] Unfortunately, other D816 mutations cannot be detected by these assays.[5] Interestingly, ASO-qPCR and ddPCR are capable of detecting the *KIT* D816V mutation even in PB in most patients with SM.[3,5,67–69] Thus, the European Competence Network on Mastocytosis (ECNM) recommends *KIT* D816V-specific ASO-qPCR/ddPCR analysis in PB for initial screening in patients with suspected SM, and BM examination, including *KIT* D816V mutation analysis by ASO-qPCR/ddPCR in cases of elevated basal serum tryptase (BST) levels or initial positive screening in PB.[6] However, most *KIT* D816V+ BMM patients and some *KIT* D816V+ ISM patients will test negative in PB (and less frequently in BM) due to low percentage of infiltrating MC. In such cases, fluorescence-activated cell sorting or laser microdissection of MC may help to enhance sensitivity but neither approach is readily feasible in routine diagnostic laboratories.[29] Additionally, infrequent cases of ISM or SSM and some cases of ASM or MCL have another *KIT* mutation at position 816 (D816Y, D816H, and so forth), or in another position, or

Table 1
Overview of the advantages, weaknesses, and sensitivity of the different tests available to detect *KIT* mutations at codon 816

Technique	RT-PCR plus Restriction Fragment Length Polymorphism (RFLP)	Nested RT-PCR Followed by D-HPLC of PCR Amplicons	Peptide Nucleic Acid-Mediated PCR (PNA-PCR)	ASO-qPCR on DNA or RNA/cDNA and ddPCR	NGS and TU-NGS
Advantages	• Simple, fast, cost-saving • Reliable • Good sensitivity	• Detects different KIT mutations at position 816	• Allows detection of KIT mutations at position 816 or at adjacent positions • Semiquantitative • Recommended for FFPE tissues	• Simple, fast, cost-saving • Highly sensitive • Quantitative: allows the quantification of the KIT D816V EAB in PB or BM • For ddPCR: works well on FFPE tissues	• Full KIT codons analysis • Quantitative results • Allows detection of non-KIT D816V mutations
Weaknesses	• Detects only KIT D816V mutant • Not quantitative	• Relatively low sensitivity • Not quantitative • Time-consuming • Needs special facilities (HPLC)	• Intermediate sensitivity	• Detects only KIT p.D816V mutant • Needs standardization/harmonization	• Relatively high cost • Relatively time-consuming • Low sensitivity and thus low negative predictive value
Sensitivity	~ 0.05%	0.5%–1.0%	~ 0.1%	~ 0.01%	~ 0.2% with TU-NGS ~ 1%–5% with classical NGS

Abbreviations: ASO-qPCR, allele specific-quantitative polymerase chain reaction; ddPCR, droplet digital PCR; HPLC, high-performance liquid chromatography; NGS, next-generation sequencing; PCR, polymerase chain reaction; RT-PCR, reverse transcription-polymerase chain reaction; TU, targeted ultradeep.

no *KIT* mutation at all (*KIT* wild type). The analysis of the precise *KIT* structure in such patients has critical therapeutic implications because patients with mutations in the ECD or the JMD of KIT or with no *KIT* mutation may respond to imatinib, whereas patients with other D816 variants would require midostaurin-based or avapritinib-based approaches. Thus, in such *KIT* D816V-negative patients, a stepwise approach can be used, at first with peptide nucleic acids (PNA)-mediated PCR to search for other 816 variants, then Sanger sequencing of the entire *KIT* coding region or NGS, keeping in mind the low sensitivity of this technique.[6]

QUANTIFICATION OF THE *KIT* D816V MUTATIONAL BURDEN FOR PROGNOSTICATION AND MONITORING OF THERAPEUTIC EFFICACY
Quantification of the KIT D816V Mutational Burden for Prognostication of Systemic Mastocytosis

Precise quantification of the *KIT* D816V mutational burden may have prognostic implications. Indeed, *KIT* D816V allele burden correlated significantly with disease subtypes and advancement. *KIT* D816V burden also correlated significantly with BST levels and age. Moreover, a cutoff level of 2% was identified that defined 2 prognostically distinct groups in terms of overall survival (OS).[67] Besides, detection of the *KIT* D816V mutation in hematopoietic cell compartments other than MC (multilineage involvement) has been associated with higher rate of progression from ISM to AdvSM and a worse outcome.[70,71] In line with this data, a value greater than 6% of circulating *KIT* D816V+ cells has been proposed as being suggestive of a multilineage involvement in patients.[68] Thus, the *KIT* D816V mutation burden seems to be a reliable and reproducible prognostic marker of SM,[5,67,72] now incorporated into prognostic scoring systems, such as the REMA score.[59]

Monitoring of the Therapeutic Efficacy of Midostaurin and Avapritinib in Advanced Systemic Mastocytosis

Published data suggest that the approved KIT-TKIs midostaurin or avapritinib are effective to treat patients with AdvSM.[73,74] The determination of the *KIT* D816V mutational burden in PB and/or in BM may prove useful for monitoring their therapeutic efficacy. Midostaurin is a multikinase inhibitor also active on KIT wild type, KIT D816V, ECD, and JMD KIT mutants. A midostaurin-treated *KIT* D816V+ MCL patient displayed partial remission with a significant decrease in circulating MC and mutation frequency.[75] These encouraging results led to Phase II studies (CPKC412D2213 and CPKC412D2201) in AdvSM, showing an overall response rate of 60% to 69% regardless of *KIT* mutational status, with 38% to 45% of MR.[76,77] Jawhar and colleagues evaluated the impact of molecular markers at baseline and during follow-up in 38 midostaurin-treated patients with AdvSM.[4] Univariate analyses showed that reduction of *KIT* D816V EAB 25% or greater, tryptase 50% or greater, and alkaline phosphatase 50% or greater at 6 months were significantly associated with improved OS, whereas only *KIT* D816V reduction remained an independent on-treatment marker for improved OS by multivariate analysis.[4] More recently, Lübke and colleagues reported a clear superiority of midostaurin over cladribine on several parameters, including *KIT* D816V mutational burden and OS.[73]

Avapritinib, a TKI that targets KIT and multiple KIT exon 11, 11/17, and 17 mutants, was first evaluated in the phase I EXPLORER study (NCT02561988) on patients with AdvSM.[78] A complete molecular remission (MR) was achieved in 30% of patients, whereas a decrease in *KIT* D816V VAF in PB 50% or greater was obtained in 25 (64%) patients, correlating with decrease in BM MC and in BST levels.[78] Subsequently, interim results from phase 2 ongoing PATHFINDER study (NCT03580655) reported that among the 32 evaluable patients, 19 (59%) experienced a decrease in the *KIT* D816V VAF in PB 50% or greater, together with profound reductions in other markers of disease burden.[79] A pooled analysis of 53 response-evaluable patients from EXPLORER and PATHFINDER confirmed a marked decrease of *KIT* D816V VAF on treatment with avapritinib.[80–82] It should be noted that the response criteria used in midostaurin and avapritinib studies were not identical.

To conclude, these data confirm the value of highly sensitive and quantitative techniques of determination of *KIT* D816V mutational burden in BM and/or PB to monitor treatment response of patients with AdvSM treated with KIT-TKIs.

CONCLUDING REMARKS AND OPEN QUESTIONS

A majority of pediatric and adult patients with mastocytosis exhibits *KIT* activating mutations. Although the *KIT* D816V mutation is found in ~ 30% of children, with 40% of pediatric cases bearing other *KIT* mutations, *KIT* D816V is detected in greater than 80% of all adult patients with SM. In ISM, the mutant is considered as the main driver of the disease, whereas most patients with AdvSM present with additional non-*KIT* genetic defects negatively affecting the prognosis. Currently, it is recommended in patients suspected of having SM, as a first step to apply sensitive and quantitative techniques (namely ASO-qPCR and ddPCR) able to detect specifically the *KIT* D816V mutation in various biological samples, including the PB and the BM. These highly sensitive detection techniques are now routinely implemented in most mastocytosis reference centers including ours. In addition, quantification of the *KIT* D816V mutational burden improves also prognostication of patients, leading to the incorporation of this parameter in new prognostic scoring systems. As well, in the era of potent KIT-TKIs such as midostaurin or avapritinib, it is of utmost importance to quantify at regular intervals the *KIT* D816V mutational burden during the treatment, in order to evaluate its efficacy, the aim of such treatment being to obtain a MR. In fact, MR of *KIT* D816V under KIT-TKIs treatment is a new response benchmark and a treatment goal, including in AdvSM. However, the concept of minimal residual disease in AdvSM remains to be established, as well as consensus definition for levels of remission. Other important questions are as follows: (1) will the achievement of MR translate into prolonged progression-free survival and OS and (2) will achievement of MR permit time-limited treatment followed by durable treatment-free remission. Finally, as stated above, a minority of patients with SM may present with non-816V mutations (D816Y, D816H, and so forth), with non-816 mutations (ECD or JMD mutants) or with *KIT* wild type. For such patients, there is still a need to find alternative (tailor-made) techniques able to quantify their response to therapy.

CLINICS CARE POINTS

- When a patient is suspected of having SM, it is preferable to analyze in a first step both the BST level and the presence of the *KIT* D816V mutation in PB rather than proceeding directly to BM analysis, in order to avoid an excessive use of invasive investigations.

- When searching for the *KIT* D816V mutation in patients suspected of having SM, it is preferable to use highly sensitive and quantitative techniques, such as ASO-qPCR or ddPCR, rather other nonsensitive and nonquantitative techniques.

- In the case of the treatment of a patient with *KIT* D816V+ SM by targeted therapy (Midostaurin or Avapritinib), it is preferable to monitor treatment efficacy by measurement of the *KIT* D816V allele burden rather than by measurement of the BST level, particularly if the SM is accompanied by an associated myeloid neoplasm.

DISCLOSURE

Y. Chantran receives research Grants from Blueprint Medicines and honoraria from Thermo Fisher Scientific. M. Arock received research Grants from Blueprint Medicines and honoraria from AB Science, Blueprint, Novartis, and Thermo Fisher Scientific.

REFERENCES

1. Valent P. Mastocytosis: a paradigmatic example of a rare disease with complex biology and pathology. American journal of cancer research 2013;3(2):159–72.
2. Arock M, Hoermann G, Sotlar K, et al. Clinical impact and proposed application of molecular markers, genetic variants, and cytogenetic analysis in mast cell neoplasms: Status 2022. J Allergy Clin Immunol 2022;149(6):1855–65.
3. Kristensen T, Vestergaard H, Moller MB. Improved detection of the KIT D816V mutation in patients with systemic mastocytosis using a quantitative and highly sensitive real-time qPCR assay. J Mol Diagn 2011;13(2):180–8.
4. Jawhar M, Schwaab J, Naumann N, et al. Response and progression on midostaurin in advanced systemic mastocytosis: KIT D816V and other molecular markers. Clinical Trial, Phase II. Blood 2017;130(2):137–45.
5. Greiner G, Gurbisz M, Ratzinger F, et al. Digital PCR: A Sensitive and Precise Method for KIT D816V Quantification in Mastocytosis. Clin Chem 2018;64(3):547–55.
6. Hoermann G, Sotlar K, Jawhar M, et al. Standards of Genetic Testing in the Diagnosis and Prognostication of Systemic Mastocytosis in 2022: Recommendations of the EU-US Cooperative Group. J Allergy Clin Immunol Pract 2022;10(8):1953–63.
7. Schwaab J, Schnittger S, Sotlar K, et al. Comprehensive mutational profiling in advanced systemic mastocytosis. Blood 2013;122(14):2460–6.
8. Nicolosi M, Patriarca A, Andorno A, et al. Precision Medicine in Systemic Mastocytosis. Medicina (Kaunas, Lithuania) 2021;57(11):1135.
9. Kim ES. Midostaurin: First Global Approval. Review. Drugs 2017;77(11):1251–9.
10. Dhillon S. Avapritinib: First Approval. Drugs 2020;80(4):433–9.
11. Valent P, Arock M, Akin C, et al. Recent Developments in the Field of Mast Cell Disorders: Classification, Prognostication, and Management. J Allergy Clin Immunol Pract 2022;10(8):2052–5.
12. Lange M, Hartmann K, Carter MC, et al. Molecular Background, Clinical Features and Management of Pediatric Mastocytosis: Status 2021. Int J Mol Sci 2021;22(5):2586.
13. Sandru F, Petca RC, Costescu M, et al. Cutaneous Mastocytosis in Childhood-Update from the Literature. J Clin Med 2021;10(7):1474.
14. Fuchs D, Kilbertus A, Kofler K, et al. Scoring the Risk of Having Systemic Mastocytosis in Adult Patients with Mastocytosis in the Skin. J Allergy Clin Immunol Pract 2021;9(4):1705–1712 e4.
15. Valent P, Horny HP, Escribano L, et al. Diagnostic criteria and classification of mastocytosis: a consensus proposal. Leuk Res 2001;25(7):603–25.
16. Valent P, Akin C, Hartmann K, et al. Updated Diagnostic Criteria and Classification of Mast Cell Disorders: A Consensus Proposal. HemaSphere. 2021;5(11):e646.
17. Khoury JD, Solary E, Abla O, et al. The 5th edition of the World Health Organization Classification of Haematolymphoid Tumours: Myeloid and Histiocytic/Dendritic Neoplasms. Leukemia 2022;36(7):1703–19.

18. Zanotti R, Bonifacio M, Lucchini G, et al. Refined diagnostic criteria for bone marrow mastocytosis: a proposal of the European competence network on mastocytosis. Leukemia 2022;36(2):516–24.

19. Ustun C, Arock M, Kluin-Nelemans HC, et al. Advanced systemic mastocytosis: from molecular and genetic progress to clinical practice. Haematologica 2016; 101(10):1133–43.

20. Alvarez-Twose I, Jara-Acevedo M, Morgado JM, et al. Clinical, immunophenotypic, and molecular characteristics of well-differentiated systemic mastocytosis. J Allergy Clin Immunol 2016;137(1):168–78.

21. Giebel LB, Strunk KM, Holmes SA, et al. Organization and nucleotide sequence of the human KIT (mast/stem cell growth factor receptor) proto-oncogene. Research Support, Non-U.S. Gov't Research Support, U.S. Gov't, P.H.S. Oncogene 1992;7(11):2207–17.

22. Qiu FH, Ray P, Brown K, et al. Primary structure of c-kit: relationship with the CSF-1/PDGF receptor kinase family–oncogenic activation of v-kit involves deletion of extracellular domain and C terminus. Research Support, Non-U.S. Gov't Research Support, U.S. Gov't, P.H.S. EMBO J 1988;7(4):1003–11.

23. Broxmeyer HE, Maze R, Miyazawa K, et al. The kit receptor and its ligand, steel factor, as regulators of hemopoiesis. Cancer Cells 1991;3(12):480–7.

24. Lyman SD, Williams DE. Biological activities and potential therapeutic uses of steel factor. A new growth factor active on multiple hematopoietic lineages. Am J Pediatr Hematol Oncol 1992;14(1):1–7.

25. Ward SM, Burns AJ, Torihashi S, et al. Impaired development of interstitial cells and intestinal electrical rhythmicity in steel mutants. Am J Physiol 1995;269(6 Pt 1):C1577–85.

26. Costa JJ, Demetri GD, Harrist TJ, et al. Recombinant human stem cell factor (kit ligand) promotes human mast cell and melanocyte hyperplasia and functional activation in vivo. J Exp Med 1996;183(6):2681–6.

27. Ashman LK. The biology of stem cell factor and its receptor C-kit. Int J Biochem Cell Biol 1999;31(10):1037–51.

28. Roskoski R Jr. Signaling by Kit protein-tyrosine kinase–the stem cell factor receptor. Review. Biochem Biophys Res Commun 2005;337(1):1–13.

29. Garcia-Montero AC, Jara-Acevedo M, Teodosio C, et al. KIT mutation in mast cells and other bone marrow hematopoietic cell lineages in systemic mast cell disorders: a prospective study of the Spanish Network on Mastocytosis (REMA) in a series of 113 patients. Research Support, Non-U.S. Gov't. Blood 2006;108(7):2366–72.

30. Kennedy VE, Perkins C, Reiter A, et al. Mast Cell Leukemia: Clinical and Molecular Features and Survival Outcomes of Patients in the ECNM Registry. Blood advances 2022;7(9):1713–24.

31. Bodemer C, Hermine O, Palmérini F, et al. Pediatric mastocytosis is a clonal disease associated with D816V and other activating c-KIT mutations. J Invest Dermatol 2010;130(3):804–15.

32. Yang Y, Letard S, Borge L, et al. Pediatric mastocytosis-associated KIT extracellular domain mutations exhibit different functional and signaling properties compared with KIT-phosphotransferase domain mutations. Blood 2010;116(7): 1114–23.

33. Monnier J, Georgin-Lavialle S, Canioni D, et al. Mast cell sarcoma: new cases and literature review. Review. Oncotarget 2016;7(40):66299–309.

34. Rajan V, Prykhozhij SV, Pandey A, et al. KIT D816V is dimerization-independent and activates downstream pathways frequently perturbed in mastocytosis. Br J Haematol 2022. https://doi.org/10.1111/bjh.18116.

35. Chian R, Young S, Danilkovitch-Miagkova A, et al. Phosphatidylinositol 3 kinase contributes to the transformation of hematopoietic cells by the D816V c-Kit mutant. Blood 2001;98(5):1365–73.

36. Baumgartner C, Cerny-Reiterer S, Sonneck K, et al. Expression of activated STAT5 in neoplastic mast cells in systemic mastocytosis: subcellular distribution and role of the transforming oncoprotein KIT D816V. Research Support, Non-U.S. Gov't. Am J Pathol 2009;175(6):2416–29.

37. Tanaka A, Konno M, Muto S, et al. A novel NF-kappaB inhibitor, IMD-0354, suppresses neoplastic proliferation of human mast cells with constitutively activated c-kit receptors. Blood 2005;105(6):2324–31.

38. Smrz D, Kim MS, Zhang S, et al. mTORC1 and mTORC2 differentially regulate homeostasis of neoplastic and non-neoplastic human mast cells. Research Support, N.I.H., Extramural Research Support, N.I.H., Intramural. Blood 2011; 118(26):6803–13.

39. Tobio A, Alfonso A, Botana LM. Cross-talks between c-Kit and PKC isoforms in HMC-1(560) and HMC-1(560,816) cells. Different role of PKCdelta in each cellular line. Cell Immunol 2015;293(2):104–12.

40. Hartmann K, Artuc M, Baldus SE, et al. Expression of Bcl-2 and Bcl-xL in cutaneous and bone marrow lesions of mastocytosis. Research Support, Non-U.S. Gov't. Am J Pathol 2003;163(3):819–26.

41. Aichberger KJ, Mayerhofer M, Gleixner KV, et al. Identification of MCL1 as a novel target in neoplastic mast cells in systemic mastocytosis: inhibition of mast cell survival by MCL1 antisense oligonucleotides and synergism with PKC412. Blood 2007;109(7):3031–41.

42. Aichberger KJ, Gleixner KV, Mirkina I, et al. Identification of proapoptotic Bim as a tumor suppressor in neoplastic mast cells: role of KIT D816V and effects of various targeted drugs. Blood 2009;114(26):5342–51.

43. Bibi S, Langenfeld F, Jeanningros S, et al. Molecular defects in mastocytosis: KIT and beyond KIT. Immunol Allergy Clin 2014;34(2):239–62.

44. Munoz-Gonzalez JI, Jara-Acevedo M, Alvarez-Twose I, et al. Impact of somatic and germline mutations on the outcome of systemic mastocytosis. Research Support, Non-U.S. Gov't. Blood advances 2018;2(21):2814–28.

45. Muñoz-González JI, Álvarez-Twose I, Jara-Acevedo M, et al. Proposed global prognostic score for systemic mastocytosis: a retrospective prognostic modelling study. The Lancet Haematology 2021;8(3):e194–204, d.

46. Sotlar K, Bache A, Stellmacher F, et al. Systemic mastocytosis associated with chronic idiopathic myelofibrosis: a distinct subtype of systemic mastocytosis associated with a [corrected] clonal hematological non-mast [corrected] cell lineage disorder carrying the activating point mutations KITD816V and JAK2V617F. J Mol Diagn 2008;10(1):58–66.

47. Dobrea C, Ciochinaru M, Găman A, et al. Systemic mastocytosis associated with essential thrombocythemia. Rom J Morphol Embryol 2012;53(1):197–202.

48. Schwaab J, Umbach R, Metzgeroth G, et al. KIT D816V and JAK2 V617F mutations are seen recurrently in hypereosinophilia of unknown significance. Am J Hematol 2015;90(9):774–7.

49. Naumann N, Lübke J, Shomali W, et al. Clinical and histopathological features of myeloid neoplasms with concurrent Janus kinase 2 (JAK2) V617F and KIT

proto-oncogene, receptor tyrosine kinase (KIT) D816V mutations. Br J Haematol 2021;194(2):344–54.

50. Traina F, Visconte V, Jankowska AM, et al. Single nucleotide polymorphism array lesions, TET2, DNMT3A, ASXL1 and CBL mutations are present in systemic mastocytosis. PLoS One 2012;7(8):e43090.

51. Damaj G, Joris M, Chandesris O, et al. ASXL1 but not TET2 mutations adversely impact overall survival of patients suffering systemic mastocytosis with associated clonal hematologic non-mast-cell diseases. PLoS One 2014;9(1):e85362.

52. Hanssens K, Brenet F, Agopian J, et al. SRSF2-p95 hotspot mutation is highly associated with advanced forms of mastocytosis and mutations in epigenetic regulator genes. Haematologica 2014;99(5):830–5.

53. Jawhar M, Schwaab J, Schnittger S, et al. Molecular profiling of myeloid progenitor cells in multi-mutated advanced systemic mastocytosis identifies KIT D816V as a distinct and late event. Leukemia 2015;29(5):1115–22.

54. Jawhar M, Schwaab J, Schnittger S, et al. Additional mutations in SRSF2, ASXL1 and/or RUNX1 identify a high-risk group of patients with KIT D816V(+) advanced systemic mastocytosis. Leukemia 2016;30(1):136–43.

55. Pardanani A, Lasho T, Elala Y, et al. Next-generation sequencing in systemic mastocytosis: Derivation of a mutation-augmented clinical prognostic model for survival. Am J Hematol 2016;91(9):888–93.

56. González-López O, Muñoz-González JI, Orfao A, et al. Comprehensive Analysis of Acquired Genetic Variants and Their Prognostic Impact in Systemic Mastocytosis. Cancers 2022;14(10):2487–511.

57. Martinelli G, Mancini M, De Benedittis C, et al. SETD2 and histone H3 lysine 36 methylation deficiency in advanced systemic mastocytosis. Leukemia 2018; 32(1):139–48.

58. Jawhar M, Schwaab J, Alvarez-Twose I, et al. MARS: Mutation-Adjusted Risk Score for Advanced Systemic Mastocytosis. Multicenter Study Research Support, Non-U.S. Gov't Validation Study. J Clin Oncol 2019;37(31):2846–56.

59. Muñoz-González JI, Álvarez-Twose I, Jara-Acevedo M, et al. Frequency and prognostic impact of KIT and other genetic variants in indolent systemic mastocytosis. Blood 2019;134(5):456–68.

60. Pardanani A, Shah S, Mannelli F, et al. Mayo alliance prognostic system for mastocytosis: clinical and hybrid clinical-molecular models. Research Support, Non-U.S. Gov't. Blood advances 2018;2(21):2964–72.

61. Growney JD, Clark JJ, Adelsperger J, et al. Activation mutations of human c-KIT resistant to imatinib mesylate are sensitive to the tyrosine kinase inhibitor PKC412. Research Support, N.I.H., Extramural Research Support, Non-U.S. Gov't Research Support, U.S. Gov't, P.H.S. Blood 2005;106(2):721–4.

62. Sotlar K. c-kit mutational analysis in paraffin material. Methods Mol Biol 2013;999: 59–78.

63. Akin C, Kirshenbaum AS, Semere T, et al. Analysis of the surface expression of c-kit and occurrence of the c-kit Asp816Val activating mutation in T cells, B cells, and myelomonocytic cells in patients with mastocytosis. Exp Hematol 2000;28(2): 140–7.

64. De Matteis G, Zanotti R, Colarossi S, et al. The impact of sensitive KIT D816V detection on recognition of indolent Systemic Mastocytosis. Leuk Res 2015; 39(3):273–8.

65. Sotlar K, Escribano L, Landt O, et al. One-step detection of c-kit point mutations using peptide nucleic acid-mediated polymerase chain reaction clamping and hybridization probes. Am J Pathol 2003;162(3):737–46.

66. Kristensen T, Broesby-Olsen S, Vestergaard H, et al. Targeted ultradeep next-generation sequencing as a method for KIT D816V mutation analysis in mastocytosis. Eur J Haematol 2016;96(4):381–8.

67. Hoermann G, Gleixner KV, Dinu GE, et al. The KIT D816V allele burden predicts survival in patients with mastocytosis and correlates with the WHO type of the disease. Allergy 2014;69(6):810–3.

68. Jara-Acevedo M, Teodosio C, Sanchez-Munoz L, et al. Detection of the KIT D816V mutation in peripheral blood of systemic mastocytosis: diagnostic implications. Mod Pathol 2015;28(8):1138–49.

69. Kristensen T, Broesby-Olsen S, Vestergaard H, et al. Towards rational diagnostics in mastocytosis: clinical validation of sensitive KIT D816V mutation analysis of un-fractionated whole-blood. Leuk Lymphoma 2019;60(1):268–70.

70. Escribano L, Alvarez-Twose I, Sanchez-Munoz L, et al. Prognosis in adult indolent systemic mastocytosis: a long-term study of the Spanish Network on Mastocytosis in a series of 145 patients. J Allergy Clin Immunol 2009;124(3):514–21.

71. Navarro-Navarro P, Álvarez-Twose I, Pérez-Pons A, et al. KITD816V mutation in blood for the diagnostic screening of systemic mastocytosis and mast cell activation syndromes. Allergy 2022;16.

72. Greiner G, Gurbisz M, Ratzinger F, et al. Molecular quantification of tissue disease burden is a new biomarker and independent predictor of survival in mastocytosis. Haematologica 2020;105(2):366–74.

73. Lübke J, Schwaab J, Naumann N, et al. Superior Efficacy of Midostaurin Over Cladribine in Advanced Systemic Mastocytosis: A Registry-Based Analysis. J Clin Oncol 2022;40(16):1783–94.

74. Reiter A, Gotlib J, Álvarez-Twose I, et al. Efficacy of avapritinib versus best available therapy in the treatment of advanced systemic mastocytosis. Leukemia 2022;36(8):2108–20.

75. Gotlib J, Berube C, Growney JD, et al. Activity of the tyrosine kinase inhibitor PKC412 in a patient with mast cell leukemia with the D816V KIT mutation. Case Reports Research Support, N.I.H., Extramural Research Support, Non-U.S. Gov't Research Support, U.S. Gov't, P.H.S. Blood 2005;106(8):2865–70.

76. Gotlib J, DeAngelo DJ, George TI, et al. KIT Inhibitor Midostaurin Exhibits a High Rate of Clinically Meaningful and Durable Responses in Advanced Systemic Mastocytosis: Report of a Fully Accrued Phase II Trial. Blood 2010;116(21):316.

77. Gotlib J, Kluin-Nelemans HC, George TI, et al. Efficacy and Safety of Midostaurin in Advanced Systemic Mastocytosis. N Engl J Med 2016;374(26):2530–41.

78. DeAngelo DJ, Radia DH, George TI, et al. Safety and efficacy of avapritinib in advanced systemic mastocytosis: the phase 1 EXPLORER trial. Nat Med 2021; 27(12):2183–91.

79. Gotlib J, Reiter A, Radia DH, et al. Efficacy and safety of avapritinib in advanced systemic mastocytosis: interim analysis of the phase 2 PATHFINDER trial. Nat Med 2021;27(12):2192–9.

80. Gotlib J, Reiter A, DeAngelo DJ. Avapritinib for Advanced Systemic Mastocytosis. Blood 2022;140(15):1667–73.

81. Arber DA, Orazi A, Hasserjian RP, et al. International Consensus Classification of Myeloid Neoplasms and Acute Leukemias: integrating morphologic, clinical, and genomic data. Blood 2022;140(11):1200–28.

82. Valent P, Sotlar K, Sperr WR, et al. Refined diagnostic criteria and classification of mast cell leukemia (MCL) and myelomastocytic leukemia (MML): a consensus proposal. Review. Ann Oncol 2014;25(9):1691–700.

Pediatric and Hereditary Mastocytosis

Joanna Renke, MD, PhD[a],*, Ninela Irga-Jaworska, MD, PhD[a],
Magdalena Lange, MD, PhD[b]

KEYWORDS

- Children • Mastocytosis • Neonates • Toddlers • Teenagers

KEY POINTS

- Mastocytosis in children is a clonal expansion of benign nature, usually limited to the skin, rarely systemic, with a huge potential for spontaneous recovery. It is a sporadic disease with some rare familial cases described.
- Pediatric mastocytosis has its features specific for neonates, toddlers, school children, and adolescents.
- In neonates whose skin is massively infiltrated by abnormal, mediator-releasing mast cells, a severe course of the disease is anticipated.
- The prognosis and treatment of pediatric mastocytosis, both cutaneous and systemic, are dependent on the age of the patients.

INTRODUCTION

Pediatric mastocytosis is highly different from adult-onset mastocytosis. The terms "childhood-onset mastocytosis" and "adult-onset mastocytosis" are widely used and incorporate both the heterogeneity of the cutaneous manifestation and different systemic mastocytosis (SM) frequencies. In children, cutaneous mastocytosis (CM) is more common, whereas systemic forms are rare.[1,2] However, treatment is troublesome due to the low availability of data on SM—dedicated drugs' safety and efficacy in children. Mastocytosis in children is a clonal expansion of benign nature—a sporadic disease with some rare familial cases described.[3–5] Pediatric mastocytosis includes neonates, infants, toddlers, school children, and even teenagers. The precise description of the disease presentations requires age at the time of diagnosis to be emphasized. Moreover, the broad age range should also be considered while investigating the pathogenesis of mastocytosis. In the worldwide pediatric population, the coexistence of *KIT* mutations with mastocytosis varies from 0% to 83%,[6] which

[a] Department of Pediatrics, Hematology and Oncology, Medical University of Gdańsk, ul. Skłodowskiej-Curie 3A, 80-210 Gdańsk; [b] Department of Dermatology, Venerology and Allergology, Medical University of Gdańsk, ul. Skłodowskiej-Curie 3A, 80-210 Gdańsk
* Corresponding author.
E-mail address: jrenke@gumed.edu.pl

Immunol Allergy Clin N Am 43 (2023) 665–679
https://doi.org/10.1016/j.iac.2023.04.001
0889-8561/23/© 2023 Elsevier Inc. All rights reserved.
immunology.theclinics.com

may suggest the need for age diversification while analyzing the molecular basis of the disease. The mutation of *KIT* codon 816 (D816 V) in exon 17, which is typical for adults, is observed in 42% of pediatric patients.[4] In 44% of pediatric patients without any mutation of codon 816, mutations involving exons 8, 9, 11, and 13 are observed following entire *KIT* gene sequencing.[4,7] In this study, specific features of pediatric mastocytosis in selected age groups were described.

Specificity of Cutaneous Lesions in Pediatric Mastocytosis

An almost exclusively cutaneous involvement is observed predominantly on the trunk and less frequently on the limbs and the head.[1,8,9] The characteristics of three major forms of CM forms, namely maculopapular CM (MPCM, syn. *urticaria pigmentosa*), diffuse CM (DCM), and mastocytoma, in children are presented in **Table 1**.

Histology and Immunochemistry

In the diagnosis of CM in children with atypical or subtle skin lesions and in cases with an unclear Darier's sign, the histologic evidence of increased numbers of mast cells (MCs) in lesional skin is used as the golden standard. Lesional skin of patients with CM usually displays at least a four- to eightfold increase in dermal MCs compared with healthy skin (around 40 MCs/mm²).[1] The use of an antibody against tryptase (standard immunohistochemical marker) and/or an antibody against CD117 is recommended.[1,10] Other immunohistochemical markers used in bone marrow (BM) studies (CD25, CD2, CD30) are not of help in the routine diagnosis of CM.[1,2,10,11] As detailed above, a significant increase in the number of MCs is observed in the lesional skin of most of the patients with DCM and mastocytoma and in some patients with MPCM; however, in the latter, especially in those with subtle lesions, the increase in the number of MCs is not always pronounced.[1,10] Moreover, it is worth emphasizing that MCs can also increase in the skin of patients with inflammatory dermatoses such as atopic dermatitis, urticaria, and pruritus, among others.[12,13] Furthermore, MC density in healthy skin varies depending on the anatomic area examined.[14,15] Therefore, it might be substantial to correlate the findings of dermatopathology with the clinical presentation of skin lesions (**Fig. 5A, B**).

Recently, dermatopathological criteria for cutaneous lesions of mastocytosis have been validated. The presence of D816 V *KIT* mutation in formalin-fixed paraffin-embedded skin and MC density greater than 27 MC/high power field (HPF) (equivalent to >139 MC/mm²) was found to be greater than 95% specific major criteria for MPCM, whereas MC densities of 12/HPF (equivalent to 62 MC/mm²), interstitial MCs, MC clusters greater than 3 (with nuclei), and basal pigmentation were minor criteria of CM.[10]

Neonates and Infants with Mastocytosis

In neonates, even if limited to the skin, mastocytosis may have an extremely serious even life-threatening course. In approximately 10% to 20% of children with mastocytosis, skin lesions are present at birth even though the disease is often not properly diagnosed initially.[16,17] Generally, in 60% to 90% of cases, the onset of pediatric CM occurs before the second year of life.[9,16] Sometimes, the correct diagnosis is established many years after the first symptoms have appeared. Perhaps that is why in some studies,[18] the onset of the pediatric mastocytosis is evaluated as follows: 55% of cases before the third year of life, 35% over 15 years of age, and the remaining 10% less than 15 years.[7,18]

Among all types of CM (see **Table 1**), the most serious clinical course—diagnosed almost exclusively in early infancy—is attributable to DCM. This is an extremely serious, often life-threatening condition as the ratio of body surface to body weight

Table 1
Clinical characteristics of cutaneous mastocytosis in children

Maculopapular Cutaneous Mastocytosis	
Variant of MPCM	*Polymorphic* (**Fig. 1**)
Frequency	Most common cutaneous manifestation of the disease
Morphology of skin lesions	Typically brownish maculopapular lesions of various shapes and sizes with a positive Darier's sign, less frequently nodular, or xanthelasma skin lesions
Location	Primarily on the trunk and the head (scalp, lateral forehead)
Course of the disease	Usually onset of the disease in the first months of life, usually tendency to spontaneous regression of skin lesions around puberty
Mast cell mediator-related symptoms	Most commonly pruritus and flushing, less frequently blistering (in the first 2–3 y) and digestive tract symptoms (cramping, diarrhea)
Serum tryptase	Usually in normal ranges
Systemic involvement	Extremely rare
Variant of MPCM	*Monomorphic* (**Fig. 2**)
Frequency	Less frequent than the polymorphic variant
Morphology of skin lesions	Typically small brownish maculopapular lesions of the same shape and size with a positive Darier's sign, less frequently confluent skin lesions, or nodules
Location	Primarily on the trunk and thighs
Course of the disease	Lower tendency to spontaneous regression of skin lesions than in children of polymorphic variant, chronic, or progressive course
Mast cell mediator-related symptoms	Most commonly pruritus and flushing, less frequently blistering (in the first 2–3 y), and digestive tract symptoms (cramping, diarrhea)
Serum tryptase	Usually in normal ranges, less frequently increased
Systemic involvement	Extremely rare in childhood, skin lesions may persist into adulthood, and systemic mastocytosis may occur
Diffuse cutaneous mastocytosis (**Fig. 3**)	
Frequency	Extremely rare, can be associated with familial mastocytosis
Morphology of skin lesions	Erythroderma and thickening of the skin with pronounced dermographism or a positive Darier's sign, brown, or yellow discoloration of the skin, usually extensive blistering (small vesicular lesions or large hemorrhagic blisters) in the first years, less frequently nodules and/or pronounced wrinkle formation in some areas or on the face
Location	Entire skin
Course of the disease	Onset in early infancy, some tendency to spontaneous regression of skin lesions with age or chronic course
Mast cell mediator-related symptoms	Usually severe pruritus flushing, blistering, digestive tract symptoms (cramping, diarrhea), hypotension, higher risk of anaphylactic shock than in other forms of CM
Serum tryptase	Usually increased, particularly in infants
Systemic involvement	Rare
Mastocytoma (**Fig. 4**)	

(continued on next page)

Table 1 (continued)	
Maculopapular Cutaneous Mastocytosis	
Morphology of skin lesions	Typically one or up to three nodular or plaque lesions can be associated with blisters in the first years
Location	No predilection to special sites
Course of the disease	Onset in the first few months of life, always regressive before puberty
Mast cell mediator-related symptoms	Less frequent than in other subforms of CM, in some cases associated with pruritus, flushing, or blistering
Serum tryptase	Usually in normal ranges
Systemic involvement	Not reported

is threefold higher in a full-term neonate than in an adult. Therefore, in neonates and infants with DCM, the frequent bullous characteristics of generalized skin involvement and thick infiltration with MCs result in high levels of serum tryptase and a high risk of massive MC mediator release.[19] Moreover, in the majority of cases, the clinical picture contains itching and flushing, diarrhea, incidents of hypotension, and sometimes anaphylactic shock. All these symptoms are much more difficult to diagnose and treat in neonates and infants than in older groups of children. In some neonates and infants, there are indications for BM biopsy because of coexisting organomegaly and high serum tryptase levels, further increasing in time (exceeding the value of 100 ng/mL).[19]

Lange and colleagues conducted a study on a group of DCM patients in 2011.[19] In all patients, the symptoms appeared before the sixth month of life, and in 2 out of 10 cases, the changes were congenital. DCM appeared in neonates and infants in two clinical subforms—large bullous and infiltrative small vesicular. The initial diagnosis was correct only in four children. In long-term observations, all children were alive with quite good general conditions, treated with H1 and H2 blockers and sometimes with systemic corticoids.[19]

Li and colleagues presented a fatal case of DCM diagnosed in a neonate (**Table 2**) and collected 10 published Chinese cases of early-diagnosed CM, among which seven DCM cases were diagnosed in the first hours or days of life.[20] In the described cases of DCM neonates, the following factors triggered the release of MC mediators: medications, food, emotional stressors, temperature changes, dry skin, infections, trauma to lesions, lukewarm baths, and use of emollients.[20]

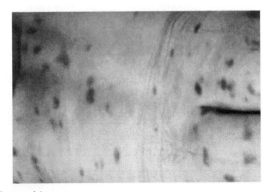

Fig. 1. MPCM polymorphic.

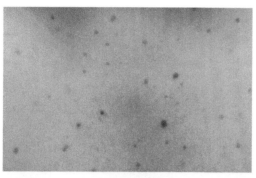

Fig. 2. MPCM monomorphic.

Of late, different cases of DCM have been described in the literature (see **Table 2**) with fatal outcomes in some cases. Alvarez-Twose and colleagues[21] analyzed the predictors for the severity of MC activation episodes in 111 children with mastocytosis and revealed that all children with DCM, $n = 9$, were hospitalized. The mean age of those children at referral was 6 months.[21] Among the 12 children with grade 4 mastocytosis-related symptoms (severe adverse events that required emergency therapy and hospitalization), the eldest child was 8 month old.[21] Because mediator-related symptoms are the most difficult to diagnose and treat in neonates, the age of patients was probably one of the reasons for their hospitalization.

Vaccines are one of the triggers of MC mediator release that create concerns among parents.[28,29] Most of the vaccines (77%–80%) are administered before the age of 2 years.[29] Brockow and colleagues, analyzing anaphylaxis in patients with mastocytosis, described one child only with anaphylaxis after vaccination, which was a case of a child with DCM.[21] Gupta and colleagues described a case of a DCM infant with severe blisters after both viral infections and live viral vaccines.[25] In a group of 94 children with mastocytosis, in which 23 were of 2 years of age, three cases of

Fig. 3. DCM.

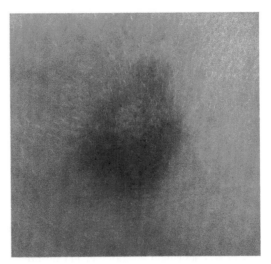

Fig. 4. Mastocytoma.

unexpected reactions to vaccinations were observed in the youngest group[29]: one in a neonate with DCM and two in infants with MPCM. In one of the infants with MCPM, the reaction was classified as anaphylaxis. Neonates and infants in this analysis received eight types of vaccines. The rate of adverse vaccine reactions in this study group was not higher than that of the general population.[29] Vaccine-induced unexpected reactions in the study group were observed in 4.3% of children.[29] Patients with extensive skin involvement and increased tryptase levels were at a higher risk of severe MC mediator release episodes,[21,28,30] also those related to vaccinations. Interestingly, a severe anaphylaxis incident was reported in an infant with low tryptase levels and MPCM.[29] In another study of a group of 72 children with mastocytosis, adverse effects were observed in four children (6%), all related to the first dose of the hexavalent vaccine usually administered in the third month of life. No further adverse reactions were observed after boosters of the vaccine in this group.[31] As infections are a real threat, neonates and infants with mastocytosis should not be deprived of this effective prophylaxis. There are also reports that may convince parents and general practitioners to increase the efforts to vaccinate infants with mastocytosis. Studies also exist, which

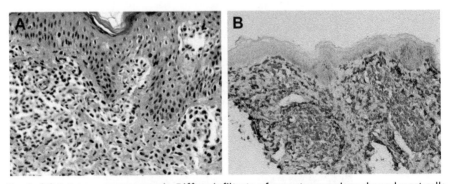

Fig. 5. (*A*) Cutaneous mastocytosis. Diffuse infiltrate of monotonous cigar-shaped mast cells in the superficial skin. (*B*) Tryptase expression.

Table 2
Characteristics of diffuse cutaneous mastocytosis cases reported in the past 10 years

Author	Time of Diagnosis, Clinics	Skin Biopsy	Treatment	c-kIT	Tryptase	BM Biopsy	Follow-Up
Hosking et al,[22] 2018	6 mo	Yes	Corticoids, H1	c-KIT negative	174 ng/mL	OK	Alive
Li et al,[20] 2020	At birth, hepatosplenomegaly, pneumonia, dyspnea, convulsions	Yes	Corticoids	D816 V	Not done	OK	Died
Cardoso et al,[23] 2020	At birth, bullous form	Yes	Corticoids, H1	No information	Increased	OK	Alive
Jenkinson et al,[24] 2019	11 d, hepatosplenomegaly	Yes	Cetirizine, ranitidine, diphenhydramine	DupA502Y503 KIT	255 ng/mL	OK	Alive
Gupta et al,[25] 2019	3 mo	Yes	H1, H2, montelukast, topical and oral corticoids	Negative	115 ng/mL	OK	Alive
Otani et al,[26] 2018	4 mo, infection	Yes	Corticoids, H1, H2, antileukotriene esomeprazole	K509I	162 ng/mL	Not done	Alive
Ghiasi & Ghanadan,[27] 2011	Hepatosplenomegaly	Yes	H1, H2	No information	6 ng/mL	OK	Died

show that transient hypogammaglobulinemia, typically with a good response to vaccines, is more frequent in children with mastocytosis.[32,33] Investing in the diversity of immunoglobulins is a more effective approach than planning to substitute them.

SM in neonates and infants is a rare but usually life-threatening condition. Numerous clinical cases of neonatal SM have been described in the literature. Angus and colleagues[34] reported a case of unsuccessfully treated aggressive SM (ASM), MPCM. They searched the existing literature and found seven other neonatal or early infancy SM cases published between 1949 and 1999, all with fatal outcomes. Huang and colleagues[35] described a case of a neonate with hepatosplenomegaly and ascites diagnosed *in utero* using an ultrasound examination in the twentieth week of gestation. The infant, with confirmed *D816 V* mutation, was treated with methylprednisolone, vincristine, dasatinib, and cladribine. In this case, MC aggregates were not observed initially in the BM. This case was published in 2017, and even though huge advances had then been achieved in the diagnosis and treatment of mastocytosis, the outcome of this case was fatal—the child died in the tenth week of life due to generalized infection.[35] Autopsy confirmed the presence of MC aggregates in both BM and liver.

Toddlers and Young Children with Mastocytosis

During this period, children start preschool and school education, which means that they start staying away from home and their parents for several hours daily. In addition, in this period, children may present or report evident signs of itching and flushing. Although the risk of anaphylaxis in pediatric mastocytosis is higher than in the general pediatric population (1%–9% vs 0.7%), it is much lower than in adults with mastocytosis.[16,36,37] Nevertheless, there is a potential threat of rapid mediator release and anaphylaxis, so children must be administered epinephrine. Preschool and school staff should be trained to administer epinephrine to children. Moreover, teachers should be aware of the factors triggering the mediator release such as excess heat, drinking hot liquids, swimming in cold water, being emotional or stressed, some medications, and food.[16] All these factors may often create a barrier that delays group education processes in pediatric patients with mastocytosis.

Abuhay and colleagues[22] observed all anaphylactic reactions, both postvaccine and nonvaccine associated, over the second year of life. In toddlers and young children, apart from mediator release episodes, the risk of coexisting food allergy other than allergy to cow's milk or egg, which increased in prevalence during the past years in the general pediatric population, starts to play a role.[38] In the United States, the top eight food allergens associated with anaphylaxis are peanuts, cow's milk, shellfish, tree nuts, eggs, fish, wheat, and soy.[39] Broesby-Olsen and colleagues reported that risk factors for anaphylaxis in pediatric mastocytosis include extensive skin involvement, significantly increased serum tryptase levels, blistering disease, systemic disease, *KIT* D816 V mutation, and previous anaphylaxis.[16] The first-line treatment of any kind of anaphylaxis is intramuscular epinephrine at a dose of 0.01 mg/kg in children. For children with mastocytosis, epinephrine should always be available in a pre-filled autoinjector, especially for those with coexisting risk factors for anaphylaxis.[16,30]

In the case of DCM, skin lesions in toddlers and young children have a tendency to be less reactive. In the majority of patients with DCM,[19] erythroderma and blistering present in infancy evolve later into thickening of the entire skin with a reddish-brown or yellow-brown color and grain-leather appearance. A partial improvement in the skin lesions and general patient performance were observed in all monitored cases, but no complete remission of skin symptoms was observed. A positive Darier's sign, severe dermographism, and diffuse infiltration of the skin were observed in all patients on presentation and during follow-up.[19,40] Independent of the cutaneous form of mastocytosis, many toddlers and young children with itching and flushing are given continuous treatment with oral antihistamines that block the H1 receptor and can be updosed[16,41] as well as antileukotriene drugs. In the case of gastrointestinal manifestation, H2 receptor blockers and proton pump inhibitors are used with equal efficacy. In a few cases of unresponsiveness to antihistamines and antileukotriene treatment, short-term oral steroids are used with good effect. In toddlers and young children, especially those with flushing, intensive prophylaxis of osteopenia and osteoporosis with vitamin D3 preparations is recommended.[16,30]

Teenagers and Adolescents with Mastocytosis

In patients with CM, puberty is quite often accompanied by spontaneous disease resolution. Patients and parents frequently ask doctors questions concerning the possibility of complete remission. In the literature, the rate of spontaneous regression varies from 29%[8] to 68%.[42] At present, there are no data that would help understand the mechanisms of this process, perhaps due to the molecular heterogeneity of pediatric patients with mastocytosis and the reaction to hormonal changes during puberty or the quality of the complex hormonal reactions; hence, further studies are needed. Children with CM presenting adulthood skin changes—small monomorphic lesions—are at higher risk of persistent disease. In children with larger polymorphic lesions, the possibility of spontaneous resolution at puberty is higher.[16,43] Furthermore, other suggested predictors for persistent disease are as follows: onset after 3 years of age, systemic disease, *KIT* D816 V mutation in peripheral blood, persistently increased serum tryptase levels, and skin lesions presenting after 12 years of age.[9] In teenagers and adolescents with skin changes persisting from the beginning of life with a possible diagnosis of indolent SM (ISM) with osteopenia and/or osteoporosis may be present. According to the recent study of Gehlen and colleagues, in which more than 8000 adults with osteoporosis were analyzed, the prevalence of osteoporosis related to ISM was low at 0.5%.[44] In the younger group of male patients with ISM, the prevalence of osteoporosis was higher at 5%. In this younger group of men, the mean age was 54.4 ± 12 years.[44] However, osteoporotic manifestations in adult men with ISM in one of the studies were 46% below 50 years of age and 73% above 50 years of age.[45] Even if the process starts early in the course of mastocytosis, it is usually not clinically overt in pediatric patients, even in teenagers and adolescents. However, Synakiewicz and colleagues[46] presented a case of a 14-year-old girl with ASM with a history of severe osteoporosis with pathologic fractures of vertebrae who was treated with steroids, hydroxyurea, interferon alfa, and intravenous bisphosphonates with limited success. Nevertheless, since in the general pediatric population, peak bone mass is achieved in late adolescence and increasing peak bone mass can prevent osteoporosis,[47,48] adolescents with mastocytosis should receive adequate vitamin D3 and calcium supplementation.

Systemic Mastocytosis in Children

The actual prevalence of SM in children is unknown because BM biopsy is not routinely performed in this group. The risk of SM is low in the pediatric population, and cases of children with clinical features of SM are rare. However, one cannot exclude the fact that the aggregates of abnormal MCs in BM, which would be the missing factor in the diagnosis of ISM, are actually present, even in younger children (**Figs. 6** and **7**). BM biopsy may predict the persistence of mastocytosis to adulthood and the risk of osteoporosis and anaphylaxis.[16] In contrast to adult mastocytosis, in which BM biopsy should be carried out in all patients, the primary indications for BM biopsy in children with mastocytosis are organomegaly and high tryptase levels,

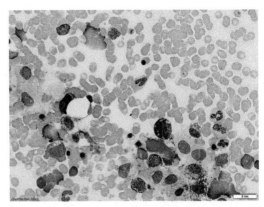

Fig. 6. Atypical mast cells in BM, ISM in a 15-year old girl.

which correlate with systemic disease.[9,17] Owing to the risk associated with general anesthesia used in children in this invasive procedure, the indications should be more precise. In addition, the detection of *KIT* D816 V in peripheral blood in children has become the basis for developing new algorithms to assist in the decision of when to perform BM biopsy in children presenting CM.[2,49] The allele-specific quantitative polymerase chain reaction (ASqPCR) in peripheral blood was positive in 75% to 85.2%[49,50] of children with a final diagnosis of SM. In cases with massive skin involvement, which might be responsible for high tryptase levels, ASqPCR detection can be useful in making decisions about BM biopsy. However, as the specific D816 V mutation is observed in only approximately 30% of children, a negative result of ASqPCR in peripheral blood should be interpreted cautiously,[16] and it should not be the only reason to give up BM examination.

Several cases of SM in children aged from 3 to 14 years have been published recently.[46,51,52] In the majority of these cases, SM was associated with acute myeloid leukemia (AML). There was also one case of MC leukemia and one chronic myelomonocytic leukemia (CMML).[53,54] In all SM with associated hematologic neoplasm cases, KIT D816 V mutation was negative, and in some cases, KIT D816 A or D816H was detected.[54,55] In the majority of those cases, no cutaneous involvement was observed.[51,52,54–57] In cases of leukemia coexisting with SM, the primary approach

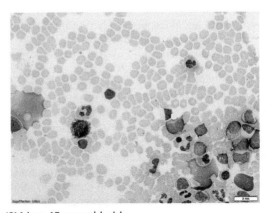

Fig. 7. BM image; ISM in a 15-year old girl.

is to treat AML or CMML using standard protocols. A 13-year-old girl with mast cell leukemia, the only published pediatric case, who was intensively treated with three courses of fludarabine, cytosine arabinoside, dasatinib, and daunorubicin, underwent an allogeneic BM transplant, but the disease relapsed 7 months later and she died.[53] In a 14-year-old girl with ASM[46] and pathologic fractures due to osteoporosis, treatment took place before the era of midostaurin, which slightly improved the prognosis and quality of life in adult patients with ASM.[58] She was treated with hydroxyurea, imatinib, interferon alfa, and steroids with poor effects.[46] Nevertheless, treatment of SM in children so far has been experimental. The dosage of midostaurin in children, starting from 30 mg/m², was established for pediatric patients with FLT3-positive, relapsed or refractory acute leukemias.[59]

Hereditary Mastocytosis

Mastocytosis is not considered a hereditary disease with a few exceptions.[2,60,61] In mastocytosis, heritability associated with germline mutations of *KIT* is extremely rare, and these germline *KIT* mutations occur in different gene regions.[62,63] In familial DCM, germline mutations such as S451 C and A533D were detected.[64,65] *KIT* mutations have also been determined in numerous cases of mastocytoma.[66] In the literature, data are available describing mastocytosis cases associated with tuberous sclerosis and gastrointestinal stromal tumors with germline KIT mutations.[26,65,67] Patients who have inherited mastocytosis in an autosomal-dominant pattern usually have increased tryptase levels, extracutaneous involvement, and a chronic course of the disease.[64–68]

SUMMARY

The clinical presentation of pediatric mastocytosis, to a large extent, depends on the age at which the disease is diagnosed. SM in children is rare and can be diagnosed at any age. Neonate patients with extensive skin lesions who need treatment due to mastocytosis are frequently in a severe general state. Toddlers may need long-term anti-mediator therapy, which may lead to concerns in organizing preschool education for them due to the need for epinephrine injections. A teenager may have to face disease persistence and diagnosis of SM. Even though in general pediatric mastocytosis is described as a benign and self-limiting disease, further observations and studies are needed to enhance the treatment options, course, and prognosis in different age groups.

CLINICS CARE POINTS

- Neonates with diffuse cutaneous mastocytosis should be cautiously observed as their general condition may deteriorate rapidly.
- Children with mastocytosis at any age should not be deprived of vaccinations because these procedures were proved to be safe in the group.
- Bone marrow biopsy in a child suspected of systemic mastocytosis should not be given up following the negative allele-specific quantitative polymerase chain reaction result only.
- School children with mastocytosis and their guardians should be trained how to apply epinephrine from automatic syringe.

FUNDING

This article wasfunded by Medical University of Gdańsk grant ST02-10022/0000701/01/253.

ACKNOWLEDGMENTS

The authors would like to thank Dr Lucyna Maciejka-Kembłowska, Medical University of Gdańsk, for providing bone marrow images and the description and Prof Wojciech Biernat, Medical University of Gdańsk, for providing the images of histopathological examinations and the description.

REFERENCES

1. Hartmann K, Escribano L, Grattan C, et al. Cutaneous manifestations in patients with mastocytosis: Consensus report of the European Competence Network on Mastocytosis; The American Academy of Allergy, Asthma & Immunology; And the European Academy of Allergology and Clinical Immunology. J Allergy Clin Immunol 2016;137(1):35–45.
2. Lange M, Hartmann K, Carter MC, et al. Molecular background, clinical features and management of pediatric mastocytosis: Status 2021. Int J Mol Sci 2021; 22(5):1–24.
3. Valent P, Horny HP, Escribano L, et al. Diagnostic criteria and classification of mastocytosis: a consensus proposal. Leuk Res 2001;25(7):603–25.
4. Bodemer C, Hermine O, Palmérini F, et al. Pediatric mastocytosis is a clonal disease associated with D816V and other activating c-KIT mutations. J Invest Dermatol 2010;130(3):804–15.
5. Ben-Amitai D, Metzker A, Cohen HA. Pediatric cutaneous mastocytosis: a review of 180 patients. Isr Med Assoc J 2005;7(5):320–2. Available at: https://pubmed.ncbi.nlm.nih.gov/15909466/. Accessed 8 January, 2023.
6. Ertugrul A, Bostanci I, Kaymak AO, et al. Pediatric cutaneous mastocytosis and c-KIT mutation screening. Allergy Asthma Proc 2019;40(2):123–8.
7. Giona F. Pediatric mastocytosis: An update. Mediterr J Hematol Infect Dis 2021; 13(1). https://doi.org/10.4084/MJHID.2021.069.
8. Méni C, Bruneau J, Georgin-Lavialle S, et al. Paediatric mastocytosis: A systematic review of 1747 cases. Br J Dermatol 2015;172(3):642–51.
9. Lange M, Niedoszytko M, Renke J, et al. Clinical aspects of paediatric mastocytosis: A review of 101 cases. J Eur Acad Dermatol Venereol 2013;27(1):97–102.
10. Gebhard J, Horny HP, Kristensen T, et al. Validation of dermatopathological criteria to diagnose cutaneous lesions of mastocytosis: importance of KIT D816V mutation analysis. J Eur Acad Dermatol Venereol 2022;36(8):1367–75.
11. Morgado JM, Sánchez-Muñoz L, Matito A, et al. Patterns of Expression of CD25 and CD30 on Skin Mast Cells in Pediatric Mastocytosis. Journal of Contemporary Immunology 2014. https://doi.org/10.7726/jci.2014.1006. Published online.
12. Rothe MJ, Nowak M, Kerdel FA. The mast cell in health and disease. J Am Acad Dermatol 1990;23(4):615–24.
13. Ludolph-Hauser D, Ruëff F, Sommerhoff CP, et al. [Tryptase, a marker for the activation and localization of mast cells]. Hautarzt 1999;50(8):556–61.
14. Garriga MM, Friedman MM, Metcalfe DD. A survey of the number and distribution of mast cells in the skin of patients with mast cell disorders. J Allergy Clin Immunol 1988;82(3 Pt 1):425–32.
15. Weber A, Knop J, Maurer M. Pattern analysis of human cutaneous mast cell populations by total body surface mapping. Br J Dermatol 2003;148(2):224–8.
16. Broesby-Olsen S, Carter M, Kjaer HF, et al. Pediatric Expression of Mast Cell Activation Disorders. Immunol Allergy Clin North Am 2018;38(3):365–77.

17. Carter MC, Clayton ST, Komarow HD, et al. Assessment of clinical findings, tryptase levels, and bone marrow histopathology in the management of pediatric mastocytosis. J Allergy Clin Immunol 2015;136(6):1673–9.e3.

18. Klaiber N, Kumar S, Irani AM. Mastocytosis in Children. Curr Allergy Asthma Rep 2017;17(11). https://doi.org/10.1007/S11882-017-0748-4.

19. Lange M, Niedoszytko M, Nedoszytko B, et al. Diffuse cutaneous mastocytosis: Analysis of 10 cases and a brief review of the literature. J Eur Acad Dermatol Venereol 2012;26(12):1565–71.

20. Li Y, Li X, Liu X, et al. Genotypic and phenotypic characteristics of Chinese neonates with cutaneous mastocytosis: a case report and literature review. J Int Med Res 2020;48(9). https://doi.org/10.1177/0300060520952621.

21. Alvarez-Twose I, Vañó-Galván S, Sánchez-Muñoz L, et al. Increased serum baseline tryptase levels and extensive skin involvement are predictors for the severity of mast cell activation episodes in children with mastocytosis. Allergy 2012;67(6): 813–21.

22. Hosking AM, Makdisi J, Ortenzio F, et al. Diffuse cutaneous mastocytosis: Case report and literature review. Pediatr Dermatol 2018;35(6):e348–52.

23. Cardoso JM, Cabral CAS, Lellis RF, et al. Bullous congenital diffuse cutaneous mastocytosis. An Bras Dermatol 2020;95(2):255–6.

24. Jenkinson HA, Lundgren AD, Carter MC, et al. Management of a neonate with diffuse cutaneous mastocytosis: Case report and literature review. Pediatr Dermatol 2019;36(4):486–9.

25. Gupta M, Akin C, Sanders GM, et al. Blisters, Vaccines, and Mast Cells: A Difficult Case of Diffuse Cutaneous Mastocytosis. J Allergy Clin Immunol Pract 2019;7(4): 1370–2.

26. Otani IM, Carroll RW, Yager P, et al. Diffuse cutaneous mastocytosis with novel somatic KIT mutation K509I and association with tuberous sclerosis. Clin Case Rep 2018;6(9):1834–40.

27. Ghiasi M, Ghanadan A. Diffuse Cutaneous Mastocytosis: Report of a Severe Case with Fatal Outcome. Dermatol Online J 2011;17(3):7. https://www.research gate.net/publication/50807942.

28. Brockow K, Jofer C, Behrendt H, et al. Anaphylaxis in patients with mastocytosis: a study on history, clinical features and risk factors in 120 patients. Allergy 2008; 63(2):226–32.

29. Abuhay H, Clark AS, Carter MC. Occurrence of Unexpected Adverse Reactions to Vaccines in Children with Mastocytosis. The Journal of Pediatric Research 2020;7(1):81–6.

30. Brockow K, Plata-Nazar K, Lange M, et al. Mediator-related symptoms and anaphylaxis in children with mastocytosis. Int J Mol Sci 2021;22(5):1–14.

31. Parente R, Pucino V, Magliacane D, et al. Evaluation of vaccination safety in children with mastocytosis. Pediatr Allergy Immunol 2017;28(1):93–5.

32. Renke J, Lange M, Dawicka J, et al. Transient hypogammaglobulinaemia of infants in children with mastocytosis - Strengthened indications for vaccinations. Cent Eur J Immunol 2016;41(3):282–6.

33. Renke J, Lange M, Dawicka J, et al. Hypogammaglobulinemias in infants and toddlers with mastocytosis - a new aspect to analyze? Pediatr Allergy Immunol 2016;27(3):331–2.

34. Angus J, Leach IH, Grant J, et al. Systemic mastocytosis with diffuse cutaneous involvement and haematological disease presenting in utero treated unsuccessfully with vincristine. Clin Exp Dermatol 2008;33(1):36–9.

35. Huang A, Fiadorchanka N, Brar K, et al. In utero presentation of aggressive systemic mastocytosis in a neonate. Br J Dermatol 2017;177(5):1439–41.

36. González De Olano D, de La Hoz Caballer B, Núñez López R, et al. Prevalence of allergy and anaphylactic symptoms in 210 adult and pediatric patients with mastocytosis in Spain: a study of the Spanish network on mastocytosis (REMA). Clin Exp Allergy 2007;37(10):1547–55.

37. Wang Y, Allen KJ, Suaini NHA, et al. The global incidence and prevalence of anaphylaxis in children in the general population: A systematic review. Allergy 2019;74(6):1063–80.

38. Michelson KA, Dribin TE, Vyles D, et al. Trends in emergency care for anaphylaxis. J Allergy Clin Immunol Pract 2020;8(2):767–8.e2.

39. Gupta RS. Anaphylaxis in the young adult population. Am J Med 2014;127(1 Suppl). https://doi.org/10.1016/J.AMJMED.2013.09.010.

40. Czarny J, Renke J, Żawrocki A, et al. Natural evolution in pediatric cutaneous mastocytosis: 10-year follow-up. Int J Dermatol 2021;60(10):1253–7.

41. Zuberbier T, Aberer W, Asero R, et al. The EAACI/GA ^{2} LEN/EDF/WAO Guideline for the definition, classification, diagnosis, and management of urticaria: the 2013 revision and update. Allergy 2014;69(7):868–87.

42. Uzzaman A, Maric I, Noel P, et al. Pediatric-onset mastocytosis: a long term clinical follow-up and correlation with bone marrow histopathology. Pediatr Blood Cancer 2009;53(4):629–34.

43. Wiechers T, Rabenhorst A, Schick T, et al. Large maculopapular cutaneous lesions are associated with favorable outcome in childhood-onset mastocytosis. J Allergy Clin Immunol 2015;136(6):1581–90.e3.

44. Gehlen M, Schmidt N, Pfeifer M, et al. Osteoporosis Caused by Systemic Mastocytosis: Prevalence in a Cohort of 8392 Patients with Osteoporosis. Calcif Tissue Int 2021;109(6):685–95.

45. Veer E, Goot W, Monchy JGR, et al. High prevalence of fractures and osteoporosis in patients with indolent systemic mastocytosis. Allergy 2012;67(3):431–8.

46. Synakiewicz A, Stachowicz-Stencel T, Renke J, et al. Systemic mastocytosis in children - therapeutic problems. Med Wieku Rozwoj 2013;17(2):126–9.

47. Saggese G, Baroncelli GI, Bertelloni S. Osteoporosis in Children and Adolescents: Diagnosis, Risk Factors, and Prevention. Journal of Pediatric Endocrinology and Metabolism 2001;14(7). https://doi.org/10.1515/JPEM.2001.14.7.833.

48. Baroncelli GI, Bertelloni S, Sodini F, et al. Osteoporosis in Children and Adolescents. Pediatr Drugs 2005;7(5):295–323.

49. Carter MC, Bai Y, Ruiz-Esteves KN, et al. Detection of KIT D816V in peripheral blood of children with manifestations of cutaneous mastocytosis suggests systemic disease. Br J Haematol 2018;183(5):775–82.

50. Czarny J, Żuk M, Żawrocki A, et al. New approach to paediatric mastocytosis: Implications of kit d816v mutation detection in peripheral blood. Acta Derm Venereol 2020;100(10):1–2.

51. Mahadeo KM, Wolgast L, Mcmahon C, et al. Systemic Mastocytosis in a Child With t(8;21) Acute Myeloid Leukemia. Pediatr Blood Cancer 2011;57(4):684–7.

52. Intzes S, Wiersma S, Meyerson HJ. Myelomastocytic Leukemia With t(8;21) in a 3-year-old Child. J Pediatr Hematol Oncol 2011;33(8). https://doi.org/10.1097/MPH.0B013E3182329B80.

53. Zheng Y, Nong L, Liang L, et al. De novo mast cell leukemia without CD25 expression and KIT mutations: a rare case report in a 13-year-old child. Diagn Pathol 2018;13(1). https://doi.org/10.1186/S13000-018-0691-2.

54. Mitchell SG, Bunting ST, Saxe D, et al. A variant c-KIT mutation, D816H, fundamental to the sequential development of an ovarian mixed germ cell tumor and systemic mastocytosis with chronic myelomonocytic leukemia. Pediatr Blood Cancer 2016;64(4). https://doi.org/10.1002/PBC.26282.

55. Yabe M, Masukawa A, Kato S, et al. Systemic mastocytosis associated with t(8;21) acute myeloid leukemia in a child: Detection of the D816A mutation of KIT. Pediatr Blood Cancer 2012;59(7):1313–6.

56. Gadage VS, Kadam Amare PS, Galani KS, et al. Systemic mastocytosis with associated acute myeloid leukemia with t (8; 21) (q22; q22). Indian J Pathol Microbiol 2012;55(3):409.

57. Rabade N, Tembhare P, Patkar N, et al. Childhood systemic mastocytosis associated with t (8; 21) (q22; q22) acute myeloid leukemia. Indian J Pathol Microbiol 2023;59(3):407.

58. Singh A, Al-Kali A, Begna KH, et al. Midostaurin therapy for advanced systemic mastocytosis: Mayo Clinic experience in 33 consecutive cases. Am J Hematol 2022;97(5):630–7.

59. Zwaan CM, Söderhäll S, Brethon B, et al. A phase 1/2, open-label, dose-escalation study of midostaurin in children with relapsed or refractory acute leukaemia. Br J Haematol 2019;185(3):623–7.

60. Tanasi I, Bonifacio M, Pizzolato M, et al. Familial occurrence of systemic and cutaneous mastocytosis in an adult multicentre series. Br J Haematol 2021;193(4):845–8.

61. de Melo Campos P, Machado-Neto JA, Scopim-Ribeiro R, et al. Familial systemic mastocytosis with germline KIT K509I mutation is sensitive to treatment with imatinib, dasatinib and PKC412. Leuk Res 2014;38(10):1245–51.

62. Wasag B, Niedoszytko M, Piskorz A, et al. Novel, activating KIT-N822I mutation in familial cutaneous mastocytosis. Exp Hematol 2011;39(8). https://doi.org/10.1016/J.EXPHEM.2011.05.009.

63. Nedoszytko B, Arock M, Lyons JJ, et al. Clinical impact of inherited and acquired genetic variants in mastocytosis. Int J Mol Sci 2021;22(1):1–18.

64. Wang HJ, Lin ZM, Zhang J, et al. A new germline mutation in KIT associated with diffuse cutaneous mastocytosis in a Chinese family. Clin Exp Dermatol 2014;39(2):146–9.

65. Tang X, Boxer M, Drummond A, et al. A germline mutation in KIT in familial diffuse cutaneous mastocytosis. J Med Genet 2004;41(6):e88.

66. Ma D, Stence AA, Bossler AB, et al. Identification of KIT activating mutations in paediatric solitary mastocytoma. Histopathology 2014;64(2):218–25.

67. Hartmann K, Wardelmann E, Ma Y, et al. Novel germline mutation of KIT associated with familial gastrointestinal stromal tumors and mastocytosis. Gastroenterology 2005;129(3):1042–6.

68. Peters F, Fiebig B, Lundberg P, et al. Detection of the germline KIT S476I mutation in a kindred with familial mastocytosis associated with gastrointestinal stromal tumors. J Allergy Clin Immunol Pract 2021;9(5):2123–5.e1.

Management of Mediator Symptoms, Allergy, and Anaphylaxis in Mastocytosis

Theo Gulen, MD, PhD[a,b,c]

KEYWORDS

- Atopy • Anaphylaxis • KIT D816V • Mastocytosis • Tryptase
- Mediator release symptoms • Hereditary alpha-tryptasemia • MCAS

KEY POINTS

- The prevalence of atopy in patients with mastocytosis is similar to the general population; nevertheless, the incidence of anaphylaxis is apparently higher in mastocytosis.
- Mastocytosis should be suspected in patients presenting with profound cardiovascular manifestations such as hypotensive syncope in the absence of hives.
- Underlying mechanisms that lead to mast cell activation and mediator release in allergy and mastocytosis differ significantly; however, patients present with similar symptomatology.
- Avoidance is the mainstay of the prevention, and pharmacotherapy options are mainly directed against the effects of mast cells and their mediators.

INTRODUCTION

Mast cells (MCs) are stationary cells and are present in all vascularized tissues.[1–4] Although their physiologic role is thought to be supporting innate immunity, wound healing, regulation of coagulation, and neutralization of venoms, MCs are better known as effector cells of hypersensitivity disorders.[1–8] MCs can be activated by various mechanisms, most often, through the cross-linking of immunoglobulin E (IgE) molecules bound to their surface by high-affinity FcεRI receptors.[6–8] Non-IgE-mediated mechanisms include activation pathways through toll-like receptors, stem cell factor receptor (KIT), complement receptors, and surface G protein-coupled receptors, including MRGPRX2.[6–9]

On activation, MCs release preformed and newly synthesized mediators including histamine, proteases, proteoglycans, eicosanoids, and cytokines such as tumor

[a] Department of Respiratory Medicine and Allergy, K85, Karolinska University Hospital Huddinge, Stockholm, SE-14186, Sweden; [b] Division of Immunology and Allergy, Department of Medicine Solna, Karolinska Institutet, Stockholm, Sweden; [c] Mastocytosis Centre Karolinska, Karolinska University Hospital Huddinge, Stockholm, Sweden
E-mail address: theo.gulen@ki.se

Immunol Allergy Clin N Am 43 (2023) 681–698
https://doi.org/10.1016/j.iac.2023.04.010
0889-8561/23/© 2023 Elsevier Inc. All rights reserved.

immunology.theclinics.com

necrosis factor-α.[6-10] Symptoms arising from MC activation have primarily been studied in the context of allergic disorders and may range from tissue-specific events such as localized itching or nasal congestion to more systemic symptoms that result from widespread MC activation and lead to anaphylaxis.[7,8,10,11] Recently, MC activation has also been studied in the context of MC disorders, such as mastocytosis.[4,6,8,10] Although underlying mechanisms that lead to pathologic MC activation and mediator release in allergy and in mastocytosis differ significantly, patients present with similar symptomatology.

In this article, the features of atopy and anaphylaxis in patients with mastocytosis, as well as the basic principles of managing mediator-related symptoms, will be discussed in light of current developments.

GENERAL FEATURES OF ALLERGY AND ANAPHYLAXIS

Allergic diseases are common in the general population and often atopic individuals have the propensity to develop reactions to allergens. Atopy is defined as the genetic predisposition to respond immunologically to diverse allergens leading to overproduction of IgE. The inheritance pattern is believed to be multigenic.[12] The prevalence of atopy ranges from 30% to 40% of adult population in Westernized nations and allergic rhinitis and allergic asthma are common in the general population with a prevalence ranging from 20% to 30%.[13-15]

Anaphylaxis can be defined as an acute, systemic, potentially life-threatening hypersensitivity reaction, characterized by the excessive release of various mediators from MCs. It is almost always unexpected and may lead to death, if not promptly treated.[16] The data about the exact incidence and prevalence of anaphylaxis are somewhat inconsistent; however, it is widely accepted that it is a relatively rare condition.[17-20] The studies from the United States suggest an incidence of up to 40 to 50 people per 100,000 person-years,[19] whereas the studies from Europe suggest a lower incidence of 1.5 to 7.9 per 100,000 person-years.[20] Moreover, the lifetime prevalence of anaphylaxis has been estimated to be approximately 0.3%[20] and there are studies showing an increase in admissions with anaphylaxis over the last 2 decades.[21] Rarely, deaths may also occur and suggested to be at a rate of 1 per 3 million population per year.[22] Furthermore, food-induced anaphylaxis (FIA) is the most common cause in children corresponding over 65% of the anaphylaxis,[23,24] whereas Hymenoptera venom- and drug-induced anaphylaxis (VIA and DIA) are dominating elicitors among adults.[24]

Anaphylaxis is a syndrome and concurrently affects multiple organ systems. However, lack of a universally recognized diagnostic criteria has long caused failure to recognition and therefore delayed treatment. Recently, multinational, multidisciplinary symposia were convened to achieve an international consensus on the clinical criteria for the diagnosis of anaphylaxis.[25] The current diagnostic criteria require concurrent occurrence of minimum two organ systems that are related to the cutaneous, gastrointestinal, respiratory, and cardiovascular systems. **Box 1** illustrates the clinical criteria of anaphylaxis in context of different scenarios. Even when there is no likely cause of the reactions, as in unprovoked anaphylaxis, when the onset of illness is acute, a diagnosis of anaphylaxis can be made when either reduced blood pressure and/or respiratory compromise are present accompanied by the involvement of the skin–mucosal symptoms.[25]

MASTOCYTOSIS

Mastocytosis refers to a heterogeneous multisystem disorder characterized by a pathologic activation and accumulation of clonally aberrant MCs in one or more

---

Box 1
Diagnostic criteria of anaphylaxis

Anaphylaxis is highly likely when any one of the following three criteria is fulfilled

Criteria 1: Acute onset of an illness (minutes to several hours) with involvement of the skin, mucosal tissue, or both (eg, generalized hives, itching, or flushing, swollen lips–tongue–uvula) AND at least one of the following:
a. Respiratory compromise (eg, dyspnea, wheeze–bronchospasm, stridor, reduced peak flow hypoxia)
b. Cardiovascular compromise (eg, hypotension, syncope, collapse, incontinence)

Criteria 2: Two or more of the following that occur rapidly after exposure to a likely allergen for that patient (minutes of several hours):
a. Involvement of the skin or mucosal tissue
b. Respiratory compromise
c. Cardiovascular compromise
d. Persistent gastrointestinal symptoms (eg, crampy abdominal pain, vomiting)

Criteria 3: Hypotension after exposure to known allergen for that patient (minutes to several hours)

Adapted from Sampson HA, Muñoz-Furlong A, Campbell RL, et al. Second symposium on the definition and management of anaphylaxis: summary report–Second National Institute of Allergy and Infectious Disease/Food Allergy and Anaphylaxis Network symposium. J Allergy Clin Immunol. 2006;117(2):391 to 397.

---

organs.[26,27] The exact incidence and prevalence of mastocytosis remain elusive; however, recent studies reported an estimated prevalence of SM to be one in 10,000 persons and an incidence of 0.85 per 100,000 per year among adults.[28–31]

Mastocytosis can be divided into two main categories: cutaneous mastocytosis (CM) and systemic mastocytosis (SM) involving at least one additional organ than the skin. Please see Valent and colleagues article in this issue on current classification of mastocytosis. CM is the main form of the disease in children with a good prognosis, as skin lesions resolve in most patients by adolescence.[32] Patients with adult-onset mastocytosis have a persistent disease and may or may not present with skin lesions. In a majority of adult patients with urticaria pigmentosa (UP), MC infiltrates are also found in the bone marrow, corresponding to the final diagnosis of SM.[26,27] Indolent SM (ISM) is the most common variant of SM, accounting for ≥80% of all patients with SM.[29–31] Rarely, there are subjects with advanced SM (AdvSM), including aggressive SM, SM with associated hematologic neoplasm (SM-AHN), and MC leukemia. AdvSM patients generally have a large burden of bone marrow MCs and carry a poor prognosis.[26,27]

Diagnosis of CM principally relies on the identification of typical skin lesions,[32] whereas SM is diagnosed according to the World Health Organization (WHO) criteria, which consist of one major and four minor criteria[26,27] (**Table 1**). Thus, the diagnosis of SM requires a demonstration of the major criterion (multifocal aggregates of MCs) along with at least one minor criterion or that there are three minor criteria on biopsy materials (see **Table 1**).

The clinical picture of SM is protean, ranging from asymptomatic disease to a highly aggressive course with multisystem involvement.[26] Symptoms in patients with ISM may be acute or chronic and result from the local or remote effects of excess mediator release from MCs, including histamine, tryptase, leukotrienes, and prostaglandin D_2. These mediators act on multiple organ systems and induce symptoms including

Table 1
World Health Organization Diagnostic Criteria for systemic mastocytosis, monoclonal mast cell activation syndrome, and mast cell activation syndrome

Disorder	Diagnostic Criteria
SM	Diagnosis is confirmed if patient expresses one major criterion and one minor criterion or expresses three minor criteria in extracutaneous organ biopsy specimens, preferably bone marrow
Major criterion	Multifocal aggregates of MCs ($\geq$15 MCs per cluster) in biopsy sections
Minor criteria	a. In MC infiltrates in extracutaneous biopsy sections, >25% of the MCs (CD117+) are spindle-shaped or have atypical morphology b. Presence of an activating *KIT* mutation at codon 816, generally D816V, in bone marrow, blood, or other extracutaneous organ(s) c. Detection of aberrant MC clones expressing CD117 with CD25 and/or CD2 and/or CD30 in bone marrow or blood or another extracutaneous organ(s) d. Baseline serum tryptase persistently exceeds $\geq$20 ng/mL
Indolent SM	1. Meets criteria for SM. 2. No C-findings. No evidence of AHN.
Isolated BMM	1. Meets criteria for SM. 2. No B- or C-findings. No skin lesions. Baseline tryptase level <125 ng/mL.
Smouldering SM	1. Meets criteria for SM 2. Additional two or more B-findings are present 3. No C-findings.
B-FINDINGS	a. Bone marrow biopsy showing >30% infiltration by MCs (focal, dense aggregates) and/or serum tryptase level >200 ng/mL. b. Signs of dysplasia or myeloproliferation in non-MC lineages, but insufficient criteria for definitive diagnosis of a hematopoietic neoplasm (AHN), with normal or slightly abnormal blood counts. c. Hepatomegaly without impairment of liver function, and/or palpable splenomegaly without hypersplenism, and/or lymphadenopathy on palpation or imaging.
SM-AHN	1. Meets criteria for systemic mastocytosis 2. Meets criteria for associated hematological neoplasm
Aggressive SM	1. Meets criteria for SM. 2. One or more C-findings are present. 3. No evidence of mast cell leukemia.
C-findings	a. Bone marrow dysfunction manifested by at least one cytopenia (ANC <1.0 × 10⁹/L, Hb < 10 g/dL, or platelets <100 × 10⁹/L), but no obvious non-MC hematopoietic malignancy b. Palpable hepatomegaly with impairment of liver function, ascites, and/or portal hypertension. c. Skeletal involvement with large osteolytic lesions ($\geq$2 cm) with pathological fractures and/or bone pain. d. Palpable splenomegaly with hypersplenism. e. Malabsorption with hypoalbuminemia $\pm$ weight loss due to gastrointestinal MC infiltrates.

Mast Cell Leukemia	1. Meets criteria for SM
	2. Bone marrow is densely infiltrated by atypical or immature MCs:
	  a. Bone marrow aspirate shows MCs >20% AND/OR
	  b. MCs may represent >10% of circulating white cells in blood except in aleukemic variant

(continued on next page)

Table 1 (continued)	
Disorder	**Diagnostic Criteria**
MMAS	Diagnosis requires presence of one or two minor criteria of SM:
	a. Presence of an activating *KIT* mutation D816V, in bone marrow, blood or other extracutaneous organ(s) AND/OR b. Detection of aberrant MC clones expressing CD117 with CD25 in bone marrow or blood or another extracutaneous organ(s)
MCAS	Three sets of criteria are required to fulfill MCAS diagnosis:
	a. Severe, episodic symptoms that are attributable to MC activation with concurrent involvement of at least two organs including skin, cardiovascular, gastrointestinal, and upper/lower respiratory systems b. An event-related transient increase in serum tryptase above the individual's sBT according to formula ($\geq$ sBT + 20% of sBT + 2 ng/mL) c. Response to drugs directed against MC activation or effects of MC mediators to reduce/suppress symptoms.

Abbreviations: BMM, bone marrow mastocytosis; MC, mast cell; MCAS, mast cell activation syndromes; MMAS, monoclonal mast cell activation syndrome; sBT, serum baseline tryptase; SM, systemic mastocytosis.

Data from Refs.[26,27,65,66]

flushing, pruritus, palpitations, dizziness, hypotension, abdominal pain, diarrhea, headache, fatigue, myalgia, brain fog, irritability, anxiety, and osteoporosis[26] (**Fig. 1**). Not all patients experience all these manifestations; however, a history of flushing is a cardinal symptom. Moreover, some subjects may experience isolated symptoms, whereas others develop a constellation of signs and symptoms indistinguishable from that of anaphylaxis.[26,33] Typically, patients suddenly feel warm and then experience palpitations, dizziness, and a decrease in blood pressure that often leads to syncope.[34] Acute attacks usually last for 15 to 30 minutes and are followed by severe fatigue.[34] AdvSM patients may also have symptoms of MC mediator release; however, the occurrence of anaphylaxis is less common compared with ISM patients. These patients mainly experience symptoms due to MC infiltration, such as osteolysis, cytopenia, impaired liver function, ascites or portal hypertension (see **Table 1**).

Monoclonal Mast Cell Activation Syndrome

Recently, novel variants of MC disorder have been introduced the so-called "monoclonal mast cell activation syndrome" (MMAS).[35,36] These patients also present with severe episodes of anaphylaxis, often with hypotensive syncope and have detectable clonal MCs expressing the D816V mutation and/or CD25+ aberrant markers. However, they do not fulfill the WHO criteria for SM diagnosis and lack typical skin changes (see **Table 1**).

SYMPTOMS OF MEDIATOR RELEASE AND ANAPHYLAXIS IN MASTOCYTOSIS

Allergic diseases may coexist in patients with mastocytosis; however, the prevalence of atopy and atopic diseases do not seem to differ from that of the healthy population.[33,37,38] Nevertheless, the frequency of anaphylaxis in SM is apparently higher as the prevalence has been reported to range from 22% to 49% in adults and 6% and 9% in children.[33,37,38]

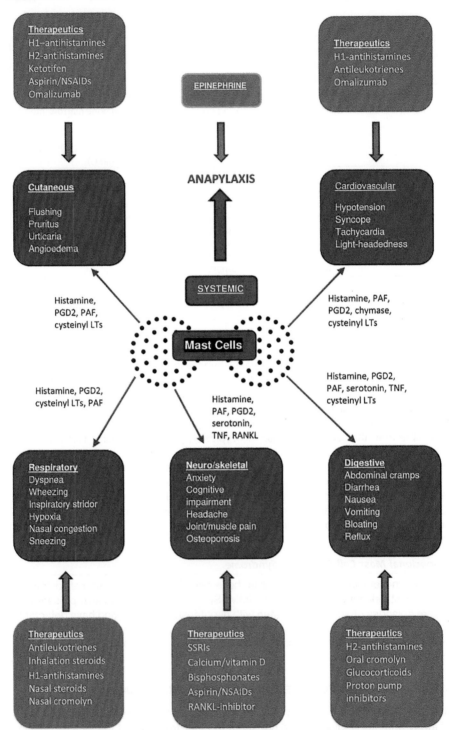

Fig. 1. Organ-based symptoms attributable to mast cell mediator release in patients with mastocytosis and pharmacologic treatment options. The most clinically relevant mediators released from mast cells and their putative effects on different organ systems are illustrated.

In our own series of 84 patients with SM, the presence of MC mediator-related symptoms was observed in overall 90% of patients.[33] Symptoms in the gastrointestinal system (GI) such as abdominal cramps and diarrhea were the most prevalent followed by cutaneous symptoms including flushing episodes and pruritus. Moreover, cardiovascular symptoms including palpitations, respiratory symptoms (wheezing, dyspnea), or neuropsychiatric symptoms including headache, anxiety, and depression were also observed.[33] Furthermore, based on allergen skin prick testing and/or demonstration of specific IgE, the rate of atopy was 30%, and the prevalence of atopic diseases was 22% in the cohort.[33] The frequency of anaphylaxis was 43% in the same study, and interestingly, SM patients with anaphylaxis had significantly higher rates of atopy (42%) and atopic diseases (33%).[33] Similar rates of atopic diseases were also reported by other studies with prevalence ranging from 21%[39] to 28%[37] among adult patients with mastocytosis.

The triggers that cause anaphylaxis in adults with mastocytosis are various, including heat, cold, physical exertion, Hymenoptera venoms, drugs, emotional stress. However, Hymenoptera stings seem to be the most frequent elicitor. A recent study reported a 28% overall prevalence of VIA among 122 patients with SM, which is clearly higher than in the general population.[40] **Table 2** demonstrates a comparative overview of SM patients and their differing elicitor patterns in three larger studies. Furthermore, VIA may be the presenting symptom that may lead to the diagnosis of SM. In this regard, one large study reported that approximately 10% of 379 subjects with anaphylaxis to Hymenoptera sting had elevated serum baseline tryptase (sBT) levels (>11.4 ng/mL), and most of these subjects subsequently obtained SM or MMAS diagnosis.[41] Another study reported that SM was diagnosed in 7.7% of 226 adult patients presenting with anaphylaxis to an emergency service, notably, Hymenoptera stings were the triggers in half of these subjects.[42]

Food-induced reactions were also reported as an elicitor of anaphylaxis in SM[37]; however, most of those reactions remain patient-reported and unconfirmed. Hence, interpretations of these data should be made with caution. Occasionally, FIA may be the initial presenting symptoms of mastocytosis.[43] Recently, a large systematic study investigating food hypersensitivity in SM reported that the prevalence of FIA in SM is at least 10-fold less compared with the prevalence of VIA in SM.[44] Thus, cumulative clinical experience suggests that the incidence of IgE-mediated food allergy is not, or not fundamentally, increased in subjects with SM compared with that in the general population.[44] Moreover, some patients with SM complain about flushing and GI symptoms triggered by histamine-rich diets, spicy foods, and alcohol; however, these symptoms rarely progress to anaphylaxis.[44]

Likewise, data on patients with drug hypersensitivity and mastocytosis are scarce, and literature is largely limited to case reports.[45,46] Incriminating medications may include nonsteroidal anti-inflammatory drugs (NSAIDs),[33] antibiotics,[38] radiocontrast media,[45] and general anesthetics including muscle relaxants.[46] More recently, two large systematic studies reported varying degrees of NSAID-induced anaphylaxis among mastocytosis patients ranging from 3% to 9%.[47,48] Some patients with SM may be at risk for such reactions; however, risk is probably lower in patients who have previously tolerated such drugs. Furthermore, unlike VIA, DIA is rarely associated

---

LT, leukotrienes; NSAIDs, nonsteroidal anti-inflammatory drugs; PAF, platelet activation factor; PGD2, prostaglandin D2; RANKL, receptor activator of nuclear factor-κB ligand; SSRIs, selective serotonin reuptake inhibitors; TNF, tumor necrosis factor.

Table 2
Major studies showing clinical and demographical characteristics of adult patients with systemic mastocytosis with regard to anaphylaxis

Features	Gulen et al[40] 2017	Brockow et al[37] 2008	Gonzales de Olano et al[38] 2007
Number of adult patients with systemic mastocytosis	122	61	154
Number of patients with anaphylaxis	55 (45%)	34 (56%)	36 (23%)
Number of anaphylaxis patients with indolent systemic mastocytosis	53 (96%)	34 (100%)	32 (89%)
Gender, male % in general (% of those with anaphylaxis)	45% (55%)	35% (54%)	46% (72%)
Mastocytosis in the skin %	68%	88%	83%
Prevalence of atopic diseases in the cohort	22%	28%	24%
Median total IgE levels in total cohort	13 kU/L	12 kU/L	20 kU/L
Median baseline tryptase levels in total cohort	32 ng/mL	25 ng/mL	27 ng/mL
Presence of syncope (%) with anaphylaxis	74%	53%	n/a
Elicitors Insect venom	62%	27%	25%
Unprovoked	31%	20%	42%
Food + drug	7% (2% + 5%)	42% (24% + 18%)	28% (3% + 25%)

with undetected MC disorder. In this regard, a study investigating patients with NSAID hypersensitivity and its correlation to occult SM failed to show elevated sBT levels.[49]

Conversely, idiopathic anaphylaxis (IA), ie, unprovoked anaphylaxis, is not rare in SM.[33,38] Indeed, there seems to be an intriguing relationship between IA and mastocytosis, as unprovoked anaphylaxis may be the presenting symptoms of mastocytosis. Akin and colleagues reported the presence of a clonal MC population in 5 of 12 patients with IA in whom there were no features of CM or histologic evidence for SM.[35] Similarly, Gulen and colleagues performed bone marrow examinations in 30 cases of unprovoked anaphylaxis without signs of CM and demonstrated that 14 of these patients had clonally aberrant MC populations and were subsequently diagnosed with SM or MMAS.[50] Moreover, a recent study reported 56 subjects of IA with ≥3 episodes/y, who underwent bone marrow examination and 8 of 56 obtained diagnoses of clonal MC diseases.[51] The reasons for the discrepancies among these studies may be due to the referral patterns.

Another distinctive feature of anaphylaxis in patients with SM is its clinical pattern and course of episodes. Anaphylaxis frequently presents with severe cardiovascular signs and symptoms including hypotensive syncope in SM, whereas urticaria, angioedema, and respiratory symptoms are rare.[33,37,52] These observations led to the development of predictive models to detect underlying mastocytosis in patients presenting with anaphylaxis but lack sign of UP. Because the diagnosis of SM requires an extracutaneous biopsy, it may be challenging for clinicians to decide whether to pursue further evaluation. The Spanish Network on Mastocytosis (REMA) proposed a scoring tool to predict high-risk patients, which is based on a combined clinical (ie, male gender and clinical symptoms of syncopal episodes in the absence of urticaria/angioedema during anaphylaxis) and laboratory (elevated sBT levels of >25 ng/mL) criteria.[52] Thus, the REMA score has been used to screen such patients and showed a sensitivity of 92% and specificity of 81%, regardless of the trigger.[52] A modification of the "REMA score" subsequently was proposed as the "Karolinska score," using a reduced cutoff level of sBT (>20 ng/mL) and resulted in a better sensitivity (93%) and specificity (94%), particularly in patients with IA.[50] Recently, further modification of previous tools was proposed—the so-called National Institute of Health Idiopathic Clonal Anaphylaxis Score—by using clinical symptoms, gender, a baseline tryptase cutoff of 11.4 ng/mL together with peripheral blood KIT D816V mutation analysis.[51]

Furthermore, previous observational studies on patients with anaphylaxis and SM suggest that anaphylaxis occurs more often in patients with SM lacking UP[33,37,40] and in those with atopic predisposition.[33,40] A male predominance has also been observed in patients with SM with anaphylaxis.[38] There are also data supporting an association between an elevated sBT levels and an increased risk of anaphylaxis in SM.[37] In other studies, nevertheless, anaphylaxis occurred preferentially in SM patients with a lower burden of clonal MCs.[33,40,53] To support this notion, the risk for anaphylaxis seems to be significantly higher in patients with ISM compared with patients with AdvSM.[33,40] Moreover, a recent study including 122 SM patients evaluated high versus low risk of developing *de novo* anaphylaxis and proposed an anaphylaxis risk scoring tool.[40] Accordingly, SM patients with anaphylaxis displayed unique clinical and laboratory features, where male sex, absence of urticaria pigmentosa (UP), presence of atopy, IgE levels of ≥15 kU/L, and sBT levels between 10 and 40 ng/mL turned out to be factors of having higher risk.[40]

Collectively, SM patients usually suffer from severe, recurrent anaphylaxis, and the various factors may influence the severity of the reactions. These include the number and location of MCs involved in the reaction, releasability and reactivity of the MCs as well as coexistence of genetic predisposition such as atopy and/or hereditary alpha-tryptasemia (HαT).[54] A recent study demonstrated that responsiveness to local activation of skin MCs by morphine and airway MCs by mannitol was similar in SM and healthy controls.[55] However, MCs cultured from SM patients showed higher reactivity with mannitol when activated in vitro.[56] Thus, there is yet no convincing evidence that the MCs in mastocytosis are inherently hyperreactive that makes them more susceptible to massive degranulation, this phenomenon, however, is still the most likely hypothesis.[54]

Hereditary Alpha-Tryptasemia

HαT is a recently identified autosomal dominant genetic trait and another modifying factor that may influence the prevalence and severity of anaphylaxis, especially in patients with concurrent Hymenoptera venom anaphylaxis or IA.[57–61] HαT is characterized by excess copies of alpha-tryptase gene (TPSAB1) and patients with HαT have sBT levels often >10 ng/mL).[58] HαT is found in approximately 6% of the general population,[62] but remarkably, it is three times more prevalent in patients with SM.[61] SM patients with concurrent HαT tend to present with severe and more frequent symptoms of MC activation rather than skin lesions or hematologic abnormalities.[61] However, to date, no studies have shown that MCs in patients with HαT are hyperreactive. Moreover, the prevalence of HαT among patients with allergies is the same as that among unselected controls[62] and the majority of individuals with HαT appear to be asymptomatic.[63]

MAST CELL ACTIVATION SYNDROMES

MC activation syndromes (MCASs) represent a heterogeneous group of disorders that may have clonal or nonclonal etiologies. MCAS may be diagnosed when the symptoms of MC activation are systemic and recurrent and MCAS criteria are fulfilled[64–66] (see **Table 1**). Three sets of criteria are required for an MCAS diagnosis[1]: the presence of typical, episodic MC activation symptoms in more than two organ systems including cutaneous, cardiovascular, gastrointestinal, respiratory symptoms[2]; the detection of a substantial transient increase in a validated marker of MC activation during the symptomatic phase[3]; control of symptoms to MC mediator–targeting drugs.[65,66]

Tryptase is the best validated surrogate marker of MC activation and should be measured at baseline and within 4 hours of a suspected MC activation event.[67] A formula of $1.2 \times sBT + 2$ ng/mL is used to calculate the minimal increase required to diagnose MC activation.[68] If tryptase levels are not available, MC activation can be confirmed by measuring urinary metabolites of other MC mediators including histamine, prostaglandin D_2, and leukotriene C_4.[69] Nevertheless, the sensitivity and specificity of these markers, as well as the minimal increases and cutoff levels diagnostic for MC activation, have not yet been established.

When a diagnosis of MCAS is established, patients should be further classified, as there are three variants of MCAS.[65,66] Primary (clonal) MCAS is defined by the presence of clonal MCs and includes MMAS and mastocytosis (systemic and/or cutaneous). Diagnosis of primary MCAS can only be made after an extracutaneous biopsy.[26,27] Secondary MCAS results in symptoms of MC activation through IgE and non-IgE-mediated processes, such as food-, drug-, or Hymenoptera venom-induced anaphylaxis. These patients have no evidence of a clonal MC population. Finally, idiopathic MCAS results in MC activation symptoms without a clear precipitating cause.

In general, a patient with recurrent anaphylaxis is a prototypical presentation of MCAS. Nevertheless, not all anaphylactic episodes fulfill the diagnostic criteria for MCAS nor do all MCAS episodes reach the severity of anaphylaxis. For instance, some mastocytosis patients with unprovoked episodes of recurrent flushing associated with abdominal pain do not meet the criteria of anaphylaxis. Hence, it is more suitable that such patients are considered for a diagnosis of clonal MCAS rather than IA.[70]

MANAGEMENT OF MEDIATOR-RELATED SYMPTOMS IN MASTOCYTOSIS

All coexisting allergic diseases in patients with mastocytosis such as rhinitis, asthma, and acute episodes of MCAS or anaphylaxis should be treated in the same manner as in patients without mastocytosis. The unique role of epinephrine was reported in the treatment of anaphylaxis in a patient with SM who was refractory to vasopressor therapy with dopamine, yet quickly improved with epinephrine.[71] Hence, intramuscular epinephrine is the drug of choice and early treatment of systemic reactions with epinephrine prevents progression to more severe symptoms.[72] Thus, all patients with MCAS or a history of anaphylaxis should be prescribed multiple epinephrine auto-injectors and be trained in their appropriate use.[40]

Relevant triggers of MC activation should be avoided. This is the mainstay of prevention; however, there is a wide individual variation among patients with mastocytosis. Hence, the general advice to avoid all literature-reported potential triggers for MC degranulation is not recommended; instead, a tailored management strategy is necessary.[73] Therefore, an allergist evaluation including allergy tests can be used as guidance to map out patients' individual trigger profiles to avoid relevant food, medication, and inhalational triggers of MC activation. For instance, the elimination of histamine-rich diets[44] or avoidance of certain drugs including NSAIDs[47] is not routinely recommended. For those patients who have successfully identified their triggering factors, the most important aspect of the management is to avoid all agents and all situations that may provoke an event. Those who are allergic to Hymenoptera venom and have a history of VIA, for instance, should be recommended lifelong venom immunotherapy (VIT), which reduces recurrent anaphylaxis risk with re-stings.[74] Moreover, before a planned surgical intervention, the patient, allergy specialist, anesthesiologist, and surgeon should discuss possible perioperative risks. Management should be planned on a case-by-case basis and, when possible, such procedures should be performed in a hospital with emergency care facilities and intensive care units.

In most patients with mastocytosis, anaphylactic reactions are usually followed by a symptom-free interval. In other patients, mediator release symptoms can be mild and episodic, or some patients' symptoms can be persistently frequent or chronic. Thus, a prophylactic anti-mediator-type drug for all patients with mastocytosis is usually prescribed for regular use or as required. At present, there are no randomized studies to show which maintenance therapy options are superior; however, a stepwise approach is generally recommended[73] (see **Fig. 1**).

The first step includes H1 antihistamines. Doses can be adjusted individually and may be prescribed up to four times that of daily recommended doses as in patients with chronic urticaria. In general, a nonsedating antihistamine is preferred to start with therapy; however, if a patient complains of nighttime symptoms such as itching, a sedating antihistamine can be an add-on option. In the same manner, the H2 antihistamines can be prescribed as a first-step therapy, if GI symptoms are predominating. In some cases, proton-pump inhibitor can be added to relieve GI symptoms. In the second step, a trial of oral cromolyn sodium is considered, if GI symptoms are persistent. The second step also involves antileukotrienes with persistent dermatologic complaints. Similarly, if known to be tolerated, the NSAID/ aspirin may improve symptoms, especially in patients with refractory flushing, by inhibiting PGD_2 production by MCs.[75] Ketotifen, a histamine H1 receptor antagonist combined with MC stabilizing properties, can also be used, particularly to treat skin symptoms,[76] and even neuropsychiatric and GI symptoms.[77] In SM patients with osteoporosis, therapy with bisphosphonates, or in refractory cases, a receptor activator of nuclear factor kappa-B ligand (RANKL) inhibitor may be effective and may slow down the process of bone loss.[78] Furthermore, SM patients may suffer from neuropsychiatric symptoms including anxiety and depression; therefore, selective serotonin reuptake inhibitors (SSRIs) can be an option to improve such symptoms.[79]

In nonresponder patients, the subsequent measures should be introduced. Systemic glucocorticoids can be additionally considered, particularly if there is a proof that the symptoms are attributable to MC activation. If the patient responds, it should be slowly tapered over a few months. Small doses of maintenance therapy may be required in some patients. Omalizumab, a humanized anti-IgE monoclonal antibody, has been reported to reduce recurrent anaphylactic symptoms in patients who do not respond to antimediator therapies[80] and has also been used as a cotreatment to allow patients to receive VIT for those who had adverse reactions, particularly during dose escalation.[74,81]

Despite best efforts, there are still some rare, refractory cases with recurrent life-threatening spontaneous anaphylactic episodes. Hence, MC cytoreductive therapies can be considered for certain patients with ISM after careful risk and benefit analysis, although it is generally assigned for patients with AdvSM. Historically, before the introduction of tyrosine kinase inhibitors (TKI), interferon-alpha (IFN-α) 2b and cladribine were the most used MC cytoreductive agents and generally provided temporary and incomplete MC reduction with overall response rates ranging from 50% to 70%.[82] IFN-α has been shown to improve symptoms related to MC mediators, considered to be safer for pregnancy; however, it has a slow onset of action and is difficult to tolerate due to its many side-effects including flulike symptoms.[83,84] Cladribine can be used in SM patients who are refractory to IFN-α and seems to act faster; however, it has myelosuppressive and immunosuppressive effects requiring antibiotic prophylaxis.[85] The resolution of anaphylaxis during cladribine therapy has been reported.[86]

KIT D816V-targeting TKIs are approved for the treatment of AdvSM and are in the clinical trial stage for patients with non-AdvSM who do not respond to optimized antimediator management. The two such most effective and well-studied agents currently available are midostaurin and avapritinib.[87] Please see the article by Tashi and Deininger in this issue for a detailed discussion of use of these agents in AdvSM. Recently, midostaurin, in addition to reversed organ damage and decreased splenomegaly and bone marrow MC burden in patients with AdvSM,[88] was found to improve mediator-related symptoms including resolution of anaphylaxis and quality of life,[89] suggesting that the drug may also be useful in ISM patients suffering from severe mediator-related symptoms resistant to conventional therapies. However, midostaurin does have substantial adverse events including nausea, vomiting, and myelosuppression.

Avapritinib is another novel TKI that selectively inhibits KIT D816V.[90] A recent phase 2 study reported symptom reduction and MC cytoreduction with avapritinib in patients with ISM.[91] Moreover, a case report described a patient with recurrent refractory anaphylaxis who experienced resolution of episodes with the addition of avapritinib.[92] Thus, avapritinib seems to be promising; however, placebo-controlled randomized clinical trials with existing and investigational drugs should be encouraged to establish evidence-based treatment recommendations in ISM patients.

SUMMARY

The prevalence of atopy in patients with mastocytosis is comparable to the general population, and the total IgE levels are generally low.[40] However, patients with mastocytosis are more susceptible to the development of anaphylaxis and MCAS. Hence, occult, or overt mastocytosis should be suspected in all anaphylaxis patients presenting with profound cardiovascular manifestations, such as recurrent hypotensive syncope episodes, particularly those with unprovoked anaphylaxis or Hymenoptera VIA. Therefore, measurement of sBT levels should be always included to the routine allergy workup in these patients.

Furthermore, it should be emphasized that there is an unmet need for the development of novel therapies to control severe MC activation or counteract the effects of MC mediators. Further research is a must to gain a better understanding of MC mediator profiles released in different clinical scenarios and explore the intrinsic changes in MCs of these patients. In this regard, the identification of potential novel biomarkers[93] to distinguish patients with severe mediator-release symptoms may provide important insight into long-term management.

CLINICS CARE POINTS

- Symptoms of mastocytosis may affect multiple organ systems, but most commonly include flushing, pruritis, abdominal cramps, and cardiovascular collapse.

- The presence of severe hypotensive syncopal anaphylactic episodes should be further evaluated for underlying mastocytosis, especially if the baseline tryptase level is $\geq$ 10 ng/mL and/or peripheral blood *KIT* D816V mutation is present.

- The basic principles in managing the mediator-related symptoms both in patients with mastocytosis and allergic disorders are similar and rely heavily on blocking the effects of mast cell mediator release.

FUNDING

T. Gülen was supported by grants from the Konsul T.H.C. Bergh Foundation, Sweden; the Swedish Society of Medicine, Sweden; and through the regional agreement on medical training and clinical research (ALF) between Stockholm County Council and Karolinska Institutet, Stockholm, Sweden.

DISCLOSURE

The author has no financial or nonfinancial relationships to disclose that are relevant to the content of this article.

REFERENCES

1. Galli SJ, Kalesnikoff J, Grimbaldeston MA, et al. Mast cells as "tunable" effector and immunoregulatory cells: recent advances. Annu Rev Immunol 2005;23:749–86.
2. Crivellato E, Ribatti D, Mallardi F, et al. The mast cell: a multifunctional effector cell. Adv Clin Path 2003;7:13–26.
3. Gilfillan AM, Austin SJ, Metcalfe DD. Mast cell biology: introduction and overview. Adv Exp Med Biol 2011;716:2–12.
4. Valent P, Akin C, Hartmann K, et al. Mast cells as a unique hematopoietic lineage and cell system: from Paul Ehrlich's visions to precision medicine concepts. Theranostics 2020;10(23):10743–68.
5. Galli SJ, Tsai M. Mast cells: versatile regulators of inflammation, tissue remodeling, host defense and homeostasis. J Dermatol Sci 2008;49(1):7–19.
6. Iwaki S, Tkaczyk C, Metcalfe DD, et al. Roles of adaptor molecules in mast cell activation. Chem Immunol Allergy 2005;87:43–58.
7. Galli SJ, Tsai M. Mast cells in allergy and infection: versatile effector and regulatory cells in innate and adaptive immunity. Eur J Immunol 2010;40(7):1843–51.
8. Gilfillan AM, Beaven MA. Regulation of mast cell responses in health and disease. Crit Rev Immunol 2011;31(6):475–529.
9. Kelso JM. MRGPRX2 signaling and skin test results. J Allergy Clin Immunol Pract 2020;8(1):426.
10. Castells M. Mast cell mediators in allergic inflammation and mastocytosis. Immunol Allergy Clin North Am 2006;26(3):465–85.
11. Kalesnikoff J, Galli SJ. Anaphylaxis: mechanisms of mast cell activation. Chem Immunol Allergy 2010;95:45–66.
12. Blumenthal MN. The role of genetics in the development of asthma and atopy. Curr Opin Allergy Clin Immunol 2005;5(2):141–5.
13. Warm K, Backman H, Lindberg A, et al. Low incidence and high remission of allergic sensitization among adults. J Allergy Clin Immunol 2012;129:136–42.
14. Wüthrich B, Schmid-Grendelmeier P, Schindler C, et al. Prevalence of atopy and respiratory allergic diseases in the elderly SAPALDIA population. Int Arch Allergy Immunol 2013;162(2):143–8.

15. Okui T. Age-period-cohort analysis of asthma, allergic rhinitis, and atopic dermatitis prevalence in Japan. Environ Anal Health Toxicol 2020;35:e2020012.
16. Bagos-Estevez AG, Ledford DK. Anaphylaxis: Definition, Epidemiology, Diagnostic Challenges, Grading System. Immunol Allergy Clin North Am 2022; 42(1):1–11.
17. Wood RA, Camargo CA Jr, Lieberman P, et al. Anaphylaxis in America: the prevalence and characteristics of anaphylaxis in the United States. J Allergy Clin Immunol 2014;133(2):461–7.
18. Worm M. Epidemiology of anaphylaxis. Chem Immunol Allergy 2010;95:12–21.
19. Decker WW, Campbell RL, Manivannan V, et al. The etiology and incidence of anaphylaxis in Rochester, Minnesota: a report from the Rochester Epidemiology Project. J Allergy Clin Immunol 2008;122(6):1161–5.
20. Panesar SS, Javad S, de Silva D, et al. The epidemiology of anaphylaxis in Europe: a systematic review. Allergy 2013;68(11):1353–61.
21. Sheikh A, Hippisley-Cox J, Newton J, et al. Trends in national incidence, lifetime prevalence and adrenaline prescribing for anaphylaxis in England. J R Soc Med 2008;101(3):139–43.
22. Moneret-Vautrin DA, Morisset M, Flabbee J, et al. Epidemiology of life-threatening and lethal anaphylaxis: a review. Allergy 2005;60(4):443–51.
23. Grabenhenrich LB, Dölle S, Moneret-Vautrin A, et al. Anaphylaxis in children and adolescents: The European Anaphylaxis Registry. J Allergy Clin Immunol 2016; 137(4):1128–37.e1.
24. Worm M, Eckermann O, Dölle S, et al. Triggers and treatment of anaphylaxis: an analysis of 4,000 cases from Germany, Austria and Switzerland. Dtsch Arztebl Int 2014;111(21):367–75.
25. Sampson HA, Munoz-Furlong A, Campbell RL, et al. Second symposium on the definition and management of anaphylaxis: summary report–second National Institute of Allergy and Infectious Disease/Food Allergy and Anaphylaxis Network symposium. Ann Emerg Med 2006;47(4):373–80.
26. Gulen T, Hagglund H, Dahlen B, et al. Mastocytosis: the puzzling clinical spectrum and challenging diagnostic aspects of an enigmatic disease. J Intern Med 2016;279(3):211–28.
27. Valent P, Akin C, Hartmann K, et al. Updated diagnostic criteria and classification of mast cell disorders: a consensus proposal. Hemasphere 2021;5(11):e646.
28. van Doormaal JJ, Arends S, Brunekreeft KL, et al. Prevalence of indolent systemic mastocytosis in a Dutch region. J Allergy Clin Immunol 2013;131(5): 1429–31.
29. Cohen SS, Skovbo S, Vestergaard H, et al. Epidemiology of systemic mastocytosis in Denmark. Br J Haematol 2014;166(4):521–8.
30. Zanotti R, Bonifacio M, Isolan C, et al. A Multidisciplinary Diagnostic Approach Reveals a Higher Prevalence of Indolent Systemic Mastocytosis: 15-Years' Experience of the GISM Network. Cancers 2021;13:6380.
31. Ungerstedt J, Ljung C, Klimkowska M, et al. Clinical Outcomes of Adults with Systemic Mastocytosis: A 15-Year Multidisciplinary Experience. Cancers 2022;14: 3942.
32. Hartmann K, Escribano L, Grattan C, et al. Cutaneous manifestations in patients with mastocytosis: Consensus report of the European Competence Network on Mastocytosis; the American Academy of Allergy, Asthma & Immunology; and the European Academy of Allergology and Clinical Immunology. J Allergy Clin Immunol 2016 Jan;137(1):35–45.

33. Gulen T, Hagglund H, Dahlen B, et al. High prevalence of anaphylaxis in patients with systemic mastocytosis - a single-centre experience. Clin Exp Allergy 2014; 44(1):121–9.

34. Gulen T, Hagglund H, Dahlen SE, et al. Flushing, fatigue, and recurrent anaphylaxis: a delayed diagnosis of mastocytosis. Lancet 2014;383(9928):1608.

35. Akin C, Scott LM, Kocabas CN, et al. Demonstration of an aberrant mast-cell population with clonal markers in a subset of patients with "idiopathic" anaphylaxis. Blood 2007;110(7):2331–3.

36. Sonneck K, Florian S, Mullauer L, et al. Diagnostic and subdiagnostic accumulation of mast cells in the bone marrow of patients with anaphylaxis: Monoclonal mast cell activation syndrome. Int Arch Allergy Immunol 2007;142(2):158–64.

37. Brockow K, Jofer C, Behrendt H, et al. Anaphylaxis in patients with mastocytosis: a study on history, clinical features and risk factors in 120 patients. Allergy 2008; 63(2):226–32.

38. Gonzalez de Olano D, de la Hoz Caballer B, Nunez Lopez R, et al. Prevalence of allergy and anaphylactic symptoms in 210 adult and pediatric patients with mastocytosis in Spain: a study of the Spanish network on mastocytosis (REMA). Clin Exp Allergy 2007;37(10):1547–55.

39. Muller U, Helbling A, Hunziker T, et al. Mastocytosis and atopy: a study of 33 patients with urticaria pigmentosa. Allergy 1990;45:597–603.

40. Gulen T, Ljung C, Nilsson G, et al. Risk factor analysis of anaphylactic reactions in patients with systemic mastocytosis. J Allergy Clin Immunol Pract 2017;5(5): 1248–55.

41. Bonadonna P, Perbellini O, Passalacqua G, et al. Clonal mast cell disorders in patients with systemic reactions to Hymenoptera stings and increased serum tryptase levels. J Allergy Clin Immunol 2009;123(3):680–6.

42. Oropeza AR, Bindslev-Jensen C, Broesby-Olsen S, et al. Patterns of anaphylaxis after diagnostic workup: a follow-up study of 226 patients with suspected anaphylaxis. Allergy 2017;72(12):1944–52.

43. Roenneberg S, Bohner A, Brockow K, et al. alpha-Gal-a new clue for anaphylaxis in mastocytosis. J Allergy Clin Immunol Pract 2016;4(3):531–2.

44. Jarkvist J, Brockow K, Gülen T. Low frequency of IgE-mediated food hypersensitivity in mastocytosis. J Allergy Clin Immunol Pract 2020;8(9):3093–101.

45. Weingarten TN, Volcheck GW, Sprung J. Anaphylactoid reaction to intravenous contrast in patient with systemic mastocytosis. Anaesth Intensive Care 2009; 37(4):646–9.

46. Renauld V, Goudet V, Mouton-Faivre C, et al. Case report: perioperative immediate hypersensitivity involves not only allergy but also mastocytosis. Can J Anaesth 2011;58(5):456–9.

47. Bonadonna P, Olivieri F, Jarkvist J, et al. Non-steroidal anti-inflammatory drug-induced anaphylaxis infrequent in 388 patients with mastocytosis: A two-center retrospective cohort study. Front. Allergy 2022;3:1071807.

48. Rama TA, Morgado JM, Henriques A, et al. Mastocytosis presenting with mast cell-mediator release-associated symptoms elicited by cyclooxygenase inhibitors: prevalence, clinical, and laboratory features. Clin Transl Allergy 2022; 12(3):e12132.

49. Seitz CS, Brockow K, Hain J, et al. Non-steroidal anti-inflammatory drug hypersensitivity: association with elevated basal serum tryptase? Allergy Asthma Clin Immunol 2014;10(1):19.

50. Gulen T, Hagglund H, Sander B, et al. The presence of mast cell clonality in patients with unexplained anaphylaxis. Clin Exp Allergy 2014;44(9):1179–87.

51. Carter MC, Desai A, Komarow HD, et al. A distinct biomolecular profile identifies monoclonal mast cell disorders in patients with idiopathic anaphylaxis. J Allergy Clin Immunol 2018;141(1):180–8.

52. Alvarez-Twose I, Gonzalez de Olano D, Sanchez-Munoz L, et al. Clinical, biological, and molecular characteristics of clonal mast cell disorders presenting with systemic mast cell activation symptoms. J Allergy Clin Immunol 2010;125(6): 1269–78.

53. van Anrooij B, van der Veer E, de Monchy JG, et al. Higher mast cell load decreases the risk of Hymenoptera venom-induced anaphylaxis in patients with mastocytosis. J Allergy Clin Immunol 2013;132:125–30.

54. Gülen T, Akin C. Anaphylaxis and Mast Cell Disorders. Immunol Allergy Clin North Am 2022;42(1):45–63.

55. Gülen T, Möller Westerberg C, Lyberg K, et al. Assessment of in vivo mast cell reactivity in patients with systemic mastocytosis. Clin Exp Allergy 2017;47(7): 909–17.

56. Lyberg K, Ekoff M, Westerberg CM, et al. Mast cells derived from systemic mastocytosis exhibit an increased responsiveness to hyperosmolarity. Allergy 2022; 77(6):1909–11.

57. Lyons JJ, Sun G, Stone KD, et al. Mendelian inheritance of elevated serum tryptase associated with atopy and connective tissue abnormalities. J Allergy Clin Immunol 2014;133(5):1471–4.

58. Lyons JJ, Yu X, Hughes JD, et al. Elevated basal serum tryptase identifies a multisystem disorder associated with increased TPSAB1 copy number. Nat Genet 2016;48(12):1564–9.

59. O'Connell MP, Lyons JJ. Hymenoptera venom-induced anaphylaxis and hereditary alpha-tryptasemia. Curr Opin Allergy Clin Immunol 2020;20(5):431–7.

60. Lyons JJ, Chovanec J, O'Connell MP, et al. Heritable risk for severe anaphylaxis associated with increased a-tryptase-encoding germline copy number at TPSAB1. J Allergy Clin Immunol 2021;147(2):622–32.

61. Greiner G, Sprinzl B, Gorska A, et al. Hereditary alpha tryptasemia is a valid genetic biomarker for severe mediator-related symptoms in mastocytosis. Blood 2021;137(2):238–47.

62. Robey RC, Wilcock A, Bonin H, et al. Hereditary alpha-tryptasemia: UK prevalence and variability in disease expression. J Allergy Clin Immunol Pract 2020; 8(10):3549–56.

63. Chollet MB, Akin C. Hereditary alpha tryptasemia is not associated with specific clinical phenotypes. J Allergy Clin Immunol 2021;148(3):889–94.

64. Akin C, Valent P, Metcalfe DD. Mast cell activation syndrome: proposed diagnostic criteria. J Allergy Clin Immunol 2010;126(6):1099–104.

65. Valent P, Akin C, Bonadonna P, et al. Proposed diagnostic algorithm for patients with suspected mast cell activation syndrome. J Allergy Clin Immunol Pract 2019; 7(4):1125–33.

66. Gülen T, Akin C, Bonadonna P, et al. Selecting the right criteria and proper classification to diagnose mast cell activation syndromes: a critical review. J Allergy Clin Immunol Pract 2021;9(11):3918–28.

67. Schwartz LB. Diagnostic value of tryptase in anaphylaxis and mastocytosis. Immunol Allergy Clin North Am 2006;26(3):451–63.

68. Valent P, Bonadonna P, Hartmann K, et al. Why the 20% +2 tryptase formula is a diagnostic gold standard for severe systemic mast cell activation and mast cell activation syndrome. Int Arch Allergy Immunol 2019;180(1):44–51.

69. Butterfield JH. Nontryptase urinary and hematologic biomarkers of mast cell expansion and mast cell activation: status 2022. J Allergy Clin Immunol Pract 2022;10(8):1974–84.
70. Gulen T, Akin C. Idiopathic Anaphylaxis: a Perplexing Diagnostic Challenge for Allergists. Curr Allergy Asthma Rep 2021 Feb 9;21(2):11.
71. Roberts LJ 2nd, Turk JW, Oates JA. Shock syndrome associated with mastocytosis: pharmacologic reversal of the acute episode and therapeutic prevention of recurrent attacks. Adv Shock Res 1982;8:145–52.
72. Lieberman PL. Recognition and first-line treatment of anaphylaxis. Am J Med 2014;127(1 Suppl):S6–11.
73. Gulen T, Akin C. Pharmacotherapy of mast cell disorders. Curr Opin Allergy Clin Immunol 2017;17(4):295–303.
74. Jarkvist J, Salehi C, Akin C, et al. Venom immunotherapy in patients with clonal mast cell disorders: IgG4 correlates with protection. Allergy 2020;75(1):169–77.
75. Butterfield JH, Weiler CR. Prevention of mast cell activation disorder-associated clinical sequelae of excessive prostaglandin D(2) production. Int Arch Allergy Immunol 2008;147:338–43.
76. Czarnetzki BM. A double-blind cross-over study of the effect of ketotifen in urticaria pigmentosa. Dermatol 1983;166:44–7.
77. Ting S. Ketotifen and systemic mastocytosis. J Allergy Clin Immunol 1990;85:818.
78. Zaheer S, LeBoff M, Lewiecki EM. Denosumab for the treatment of osteoporosis. Expert Opin Drug Metab Toxicol 2015;11:461–70.
79. Moura DS, Georgin-Lavialle S, Gaillard R, et al. Neuropsychological features of adult mastocytosis. Immunol Allergy Clin North Am 2014;34(2):407–22.
80. Jendoubi F, Gaudenzio N, Gallini A, et al. Omalizumab in the treatment of adult patients with mastocytosis: a systematic review. Clin Exp Allergy 2020;50(6):654–61.
81. Kontou-Fili K, Filis CI. Prolonged high-dose omalizumab is required to control reactions to venom immunotherapy in mastocytosis. Allergy 2009;64:1384–5.
82. Valent P, Sperr WR, Akin C. How I treat patients with advanced systemic mastocytosis. Blood 2010;116:5812–7.
83. Kluin-Nelemans HC, Jansen JH, Breukelman H, et al. Response to interferon alfa-2b in a patient with systemic mastocytosis. N Engl J Med 1992;326:619–23.
84. Butterfield JH. Response of severe systemic mastocytosis to interferon alpha. Br J Dermatol 1998;138:489–95.
85. Tefferi A, Li CY, Butterfield JH, et al. Treatment of systemic mast-cell disease with cladribine. N Engl J Med 2001;344:307–9.
86. Wimazal F, Geissler P, Shnawa P, et al. Severe life-threatening or disabling anaphylaxis in patients with systemic mastocytosis: a single-center experience. Int Arch Allergy Immunol 2012;157(4):399–405.
87. Akin C, Arock M, Valent P. Tyrosine kinase inhibitors for the treatment of indolent systemic mastocytosis: Are we there yet? J Allergy Clin Immunol 2022 Jun;149(6):1912–8.
88. Gotlib J, Kluin-Nelemans HC, George TI, et al. Efficacy and safety of midostaurin in advanced systemic mastocytosis. N Engl J Med 2016;374(26):2530–41.
89. Hartmann K, Gotlib J, Akin C, et al. Midostaurin improves quality of life and mediator-related symptoms in advanced systemic mastocytosis. J Allergy Clin Immunol 2020;146(2):356–66.
90. Gilreath JA, Tchertanov L, Deininger MW. Novel approaches to treating advanced systemic mastocytosis. Clin Pharmacol 2019;11:77–92.

91. Akin C, Elberink HO, Gotlib J, et al. PIONEER: a randomized, double-blind, placebo-controlled, phase 2 study of avapritinib in patients with indolent or smoldering systemic mastocytosis (SM) with symptoms inadequately controlled by standard therapy. J Allergy Clin Immunol 2020;145(2):AB336.

92. Kudlaty E, Perez M, Stein BL, et al. Systemic mastocytosis with an associated hematologic neoplasm complicated by recurrent anaphylaxis: prompt resolution of anaphylaxis with the addition of avapritinib. J Allergy Clin Immunol Pract 2021; 9(6):2534–6.

93. Gulen T, Teufelberger A, Ekoff M, et al. Distinct plasma biomarkers confirm the diagnosis of mastocytosis and identify increased risk of anaphylaxis. J Allergy Clin Immunol 2021;148(3):889–94.

Drug and Venom Allergy in Mastocytosis

Matthew P. Giannetti, MD[a,b,*],
Jennifer Nicoloro-SantaBarbara, PhD[b,c], Grace Godwin, BA[a],
Julia Middlesworth, BS[a], Andrew Espeland, BS, BA[a],
Mariana C. Castells, MD, PhD[a,b]

KEYWORDS

- Nonsteroidal antiinflammatory drugs (NSAIDs) • Antibiotics • Vaccines
- Perioperative anaphylaxis

KEY POINTS

- Hymenoptera stings may cause anaphylaxis in up to 25% of patients with mastocytosis, and lifelong venom immunotherapy is recommended for immunoglobulin E sensitization.
- Nonsteroidal antiinflammaotry drugs, opioids, radio contrast media, vancomycin, and quinolones may cause anaphylaxis in patients with clonal mast cell disorders, and there is a need to identify patients at risk.
- Premedications protect patients with mastocytosis during surgical invasive procedures and contrast media exposure.

INTRODUCTION

"Doctor, I cannot take any pain medications. I have mastocytosis. –Have you ever had a reaction to aspirin, ibuprofen or other similar medications? – I have never tried since I was diagnosed of skin mastocytosis when I was 20 and now I have arthritis and need pain medication. What can I take?" The patient's medical records present a wide list of unverified allergies and the patient is labeled "Allergy to all NSAIDS."

This is a common scenario for health care providers taking care of patients with cutaneous and systemic mastocytosis. How to address potential reactions to drugs in mastocytosis is a challenging field that has not been standardized. How to best protect patients when exposed to medications with potential for mast cell activation has not reached universal consensus. Patients with mastocytosis have a disproportionate

[a] Division of Allergy and Clinical Immunology, Brigham and Women's Hospital, 41 Avenue Louis Pasteur, Alumni Hall, Room 303, Boston, MA 02115, USA; [b] Harvard Medical School, 41 Avenue Louis Pasteur, Alumni Hall, Room 303, Boston, MA 02115, USA; [c] Department of Psychiatry, Brigham and Women's Hospital, 41 Avenue Louis Pasteur, Alumni Hall, Room 303, Boston, MA 02115, USA
* Corresponding author. Division of Allergy and Clinical Immunology, Brigham and Women's Hospital, 60 Fenwood Road, Hale Building for Transformational Medicine, 5th floor, Boston, MA 02132.
E-mail address: mgiannetti@bwh.harvard.edu

Immunol Allergy Clin N Am 43 (2023) 699–710
https://doi.org/10.1016/j.iac.2023.04.002
0889-8561/23/© 2023 Elsevier Inc. All rights reserved.

increase in the number of mast cells in the skin, bone marrow, and other organs and carry activating KIT mutations, placing them at risk for reactions when exposed to drugs known to activate mast cells through immunoglobulin E (IgE) and non-IgE mechanisms. Increased frequency in Hymenoptera venom–induced anaphylaxis is reported in patients with mastocytosis and can be the initial presentation leading to the diagnosis; this is often missed by providers if paired tryptase levels are not obtained. Duplications of TPSAB1 genes that increase baseline serum tryptase levels are more frequent in patients with mastocytosis than in the general population, adding risk for mast cell activation events including anaphylaxis. The true incidence of drug allergy and hypersensitivity in patients with mastocytosis is not known, and fear of mast cell activation deprives adult and pediatric patients of important medications such as nonsteroidal anti-inflammatory drugs (NSAIDs), opioids, vaccines, and contrast media among others. We provide here updated information on current approaches to drug and Hymenoptera allergy in mastocytosis to spur personalized care.

VENOM HYPERSENSITIVITY

More than half of adults worldwide (56%–94%) have been stung by a Hymenoptera insect in their lifetime,[1] with 0.3% to 8.9% developing systemic symptoms after sting (anaphylaxis).[1,2] Of those developing a Hymenoptera-induced systemic reaction, 1% to 7.9% have a clonal mast cell disease.[3] In fact, Hymenoptera insect sting is the most common trigger for anaphylaxis in mastocytosis.[1–3] The incidence of Hymenoptera-induced systemic reactions (or anaphylaxis) in individuals with systemic mastocytosis is far greater and more severe than what is observed in the general population,[4,5] with estimates as high as 20% to 50%.[6–9] This increase in severity and incidence may be due to IgE-mediated and/or non–IgE-mediated activation of mast cells among individuals with mast cell disorders (**Fig. 1**). Fatalities have been reported in several cases.[10]

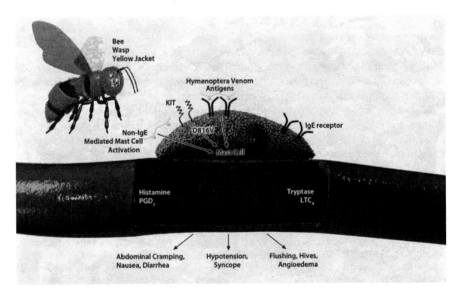

Fig. 1. Mast cell defects that may collectively lead to increased risk for anaphylaxis in response to Hymenoptera venom in patients with clonal mast cell disease. LTC_4, leukotriene C4; PGD_2, prostaglandin D2. (*From* Castells MC, Hornick JL, Akin C. Anaphylaxis after hymenoptera sting: is it venom allergy, a clonal disorder, or both? J Allergy Clin Immunol Pract. 2015;3(3):350-355.)

Although Hymenoptera-induced anaphylaxis can occur in all variants of mastocytosis, individuals with indolent systemic mastocytosis and IgE levels greater than or equal to 15 kU/L[11] without skin lesions are at greatest risk.[9,12] These individuals tend to be men with lower basal serum tryptase levels.[2,13] Hymenoptera-induced anaphylaxis in mastocytosis has unique clinical features characterized by cardiovascular vasodilatory-related symptoms (eg, dizziness, hypotension, and loss of consciousness).[1,2,14]

Because of the potential severity, evaluation of patients with a pertinent history is an important intervention. Skin testing and serum-specific IgE evaluation should occur a minimum of 4 to 6 weeks after venom exposure[15–17] and is safe in individuals with systemic mastocytosis.[18] In those without detectable IgE sensitization, repeat evaluation in 6 months since prolonged lack of skin mast cell reactivity has been observed after systemic mast cell activation and natural desensitization. Any patient with evidence of IgE sensitization and a relevant clinical history should undergo venom immunotherapy (VIT).

VIT can be challenging in patients with clonal mast cell activation disorders, as there is an elevated risk of adverse reactions during the build-up phase of the vaccination process when increasing doses are administered and can trigger anaphylaxis.[19] Between 18.9% and 34% of individuals with mastocytosis report experiencing side effects from VIT,[20] with most of them experiencing a reaction during the initial build-up phase when the immune mechanisms leading to tolerance have not been established.[21] Patients with mastocytosis can react to very small amount of VIT allergens with systemic mast cell activation including hypotension and protecting them has been difficult until recently, when anti-IgE has become available, although there is no current Food and Drug Administration indication. Omalizumab, anti-IgE, has shown to reduce the risk of severe reactions,[19] but many individuals discontinue VIT due to severe adverse reactions and safety concerns.[22] Ultrarush 3-day protocols for VIT have been developed, and although less time consuming as compared with classic VIT, the rate of adverse reactions has been reported to be similar to that of conventional VIT. An ultrarush 6-hour venom desensitization protocol for patients with Hymenoptera venom anaphylaxis was developed more recently, which safely achieved maintenance doses in individuals with clonal mast cell disorders with and without omalizumab.[22] The protocol is graphically displayed in **Table 1**. This rapid induction of tolerance can provide protection to high-risk populations with immediate needs such as beekeepers and outdoors workers. Auto-injectable epinephrine devices need to be available to all patients with Hymenoptera venom–reactive mastocytosis with yearly education on technique and indications.

NONSTEROIDAL ANTIINFLAMMATORY DRUGS

Patients with mastocytosis have a higher risk of adverse reactions to NSAIDs compared with the general population, and NSAIDs can trigger anaphylaxis[23–25] and hypotensive syncope.[26,27]

There are few studies describing the prevalence of NSAID hypersensitivity in this population. The largest study retrospectively reviewed 641 children and adults from Spain and Portugal and included adults with all variants of mastocytosis and children with cutaneous and systemic mastocytosis. NSAID hypersensitivity was diagnosed based on history with confirmatory challenges performed in 48/51 (94%) of adults with reported intolerance. The study reported that 87% of adults and 91% of children are tolerant of NSAIDs.[23] Patients with a reported adverse history of NSAIDs most often reacted to a single agent.[23] Further, most patients with a history of adverse reactions to NSAIDs tolerated acetaminophen and paracetamol.

Table 1
Hymenoptera venom ultrarush desensitization protocol for use in patients with clonal mast cell disorders

Step	Time (min)	Dilution	Concentration (μg)/mL	Volume (mL) subcutaneously	Dose (μg)	Cumulative dose (μg)
1	0	1:1000	0.3	0.2	0.06	0.1
2	30	1:1000	0.3	0.4	0.12	0.2
3	60	1:1000	0.3	0.8	0.24	0.4
4	90	1:100	3	0.2	0.6	1.0
5	120	1:100	3	0.4	1.2	2.2
6	150	1:100	3	0.8	2.4	4.6
7	180	1:10	30	0.2	6	10.6
8	210	1:10	30	0.4	12	22.6
9	240	1:10	30	0.8	24	46.6
10	270	1:1	300	0.1	30	76.6
II	300	1:1	300	0.25	75	151.6
12	330	1:1	300	0.5	150	301.6

Three dilutions of standard venom extract are created (1:1000, 1:100, 1:10). Each dose is administered in 30-min intervals. The first maintenance dose was administered 2 wk after desensitization, followed by once-monthly injections.

From Giannetti M, Silver J, Hufdhi R, Castells M. One-day ultrarush desensitization for Hymenoptera venom anaphylaxis in patients with and without mast cell disorders with adjuvant omalizumab. *J Allergy Clin Immunol Pract.* 2020;8(4):1431-1435.e3.

The pathophysiology of adverse reactions to NSAIDs is unknown, and direct cyclooxygenase 1 inhibition with shunting to leukotrienes production has been suggested, and an increase in mast cell mediators including prostaglandin, leukotriene, and histamine during adverse reactions has been observed.[28] Whether new mast cell receptors expressed by KITD816V-mutated mast cells such as Mas-related G protein–coupled receptor X2 (MRGPRX2) can be the target of NSAIDs is not known. NSAIDs may also act as anaphylaxis cofactors and lower the threshold for systemic reactions.[26] One case report describes a patient with systemic mastocytosis and oral allergy syndrome to carrot. Ingestion of acetylsalicylic acid before carrot consumption led to anaphylaxis.[29]

NSAIDs block PDG2 generation and represent important tools to control symptoms in patients with mastocytosis.[30] Patients with flushing and/or overproduction of prostaglandin metabolites may benefit from therapy with Aspirin, which should be started in a controlled clinical setting at low dose and increased as tolerated to doses recommended for patients with aspirin exacerbated respiratory disease.[24,31] Aspirin-intolerant patients may benefit from desensitization and requires the proper clinical setting, as hypotension and severe anaphylaxis have been reported.[32]

Addressing NSAID tolerance is important in mastocytosis to prevent unnecessary avoidance and the potential overuse of other pain medications such as opioids. Delabeling should be done at each patient visit, as previously tolerant patients may become intolerant. Protecting intolerant patients should be done by specific labeling in medical charts.

RADIOCONTRAST MEDIA

In the general population, adverse reactions to radiocontrast media (RCMs) are rare and occur in approximately 0.7% of infusions with nonionic contrast media.[33]

Although there is limited evidence to determine the risk in patients with mastocytosis,[30] anecdotal reports indicate both ionic and nonionic contrast media can induce severe reactions with hypotension and cardiovascular collapse.

One study with a cohort of 120 patients with mastocytosis (both adult and pediatric) found that RCMs were a trigger for anaphylaxis in 2 adult patients although severity of reactions were not specifically described.[7,26] Two studies from the Spanish Mastocytosis Center describe 50 adult and pediatric patients with mastocytosis or mast cell activation episodes, and there were no reported reactions to RCM.[34,35] More importantly, a large European cohort of patients with immediate and nonimmediate reactions to RCM included 220 patients, none of whom had a clonal mast cell disorder.[36] Case reports demonstrate the occurrence of severe anaphylaxis,[37] and tryptase elevations can provide evidence of systemic mast cell activation through non-IgE mechanisms. Premedications may protect mastocytosis patients, and one study reported tolerance of identical medication (iohexol 300) after premedication with systemic prednisone and diphenhydramine.[37]

There are no evidence-based data supporting empirical premedications, and the current recommendations are medical center specific. Whether the use of premedications protects patients from systemic mast cell activation is unknown, and there is consensus that all patients with previous reactions should be premedicated. The use of steroids should be limited in pediatric patients and nonsedating antihistamines should be preferred based on limited data on desensitized patients.[30,38,39]

OPIOIDS

Opioids are often reported to cause adverse drug reactions in patients with mastocytosis but there are no controlled studies indicating the prevalence and the specificity, and most centers recommend avoidance as a general rule. Mastocytosis patients in need of pain medications during major surgery, bone fractures, or other pain-inducing conditions need to be provided with specific recommendations or alternatives. There are few studies that address the mechanism of adverse reactions but both IgE-mediated and non–IgE-mediated mechanisms are possible, and activation of the new MRGPRX2 receptor may occur.

In vitro data show opioids have a concentration-dependent ability to elicit both histamine and tryptase secretion from mast cells[7]; this is observed with morphine, buprenorphine, codeine, and meperidine. This ability may be related to the chemical composition of the drug, as fentanyl and synthetic opioids seem to induce less mediator release.[40] Morphine is capable of inducing histamine and tryptase release but not the generation of prostaglandin metabolites. Synthetic opioids did not induce the release of histamine or tryptase from in vitro mast cells. Less systemic vasodilation has been noted with synthetic opioids, likely secondary to decreased histamine release.[41] Overall, synthetic opioids are thought to have less potential to activate mast cells and preferred wherever possible but should be limited due to potential addiction. NSAIDs, which are well tolerated by most of the patients with mastocytosis should be the first line of pain medications.

PERIOPERATIVE ANAPHYLAXIS

Procedures involving anesthesia may pose a risk to patients with mastocytosis, as the incidence of mast cell mediator release symptoms and anaphylaxis is higher compared with the general population.[42,43] Several studies have examined adverse reactions and anaphylaxis in patients with clonal mast cell disorders in the perioperative setting. The largest study analyzed 501 pediatric and adult patients across

726 procedures.[43] The study identified an increased risk of anaphylaxis in both children and adults (2% and 0.4%, respectively) with major surgery and general anesthesia as statistically significant risk factors. Interestingly, most cases did not implicate a specific medication, and patients often tolerated the same anesthesia if administered under premedication.[43,44]

The mechanisms for increased rate of adverse reactions are likely multifactorial. Ketamine, propofol, and muscle relaxants can activate human mast cells and directly cause mediator release.[45,46] Other compounds may activate mast cells via the unique cationic G protein–coupled receptor, MRPGRX2.[47] Finally, antibiotics and other compounds may trigger adverse reactions in an IgE-dependent manner.[7,48]

Because of increased risk of perioperative symptoms, a careful evaluation before any invasive procedure should be done; this may include a detailed history including prior procedures and adverse reactions including anaphylaxis.

In the event of perioperative mast cell release symptoms and anaphylaxis, the retrospective identification of the culprit drug will help make recommendations for avoidance and protect patients in future exposures. **Fig. 2** reviews the acute management and subsequent evaluation of perioperative hypersensitivity. If no culprit is identified, premedication with H_1-antihistamines and systemic corticosteroids and changing all the drugs used in the previous event has reduced the incidence of mast cell mediator release in further procedures as seen in other clinical contexts.[30] No placebo-controlled trials evaluating the efficacy of premedication during anesthesia have been done, and premedication is recommended for all patients with previous reactions, high mast cell burden, and advanced diseases.[26]

ANTIBIOTICS

Patients with systemic mastocytosis are thought to be at a higher risk of adverse reactions from antibiotics although studies involving provocation challenges are not available to identify reactors, and systematic skin testing has not been done to assess

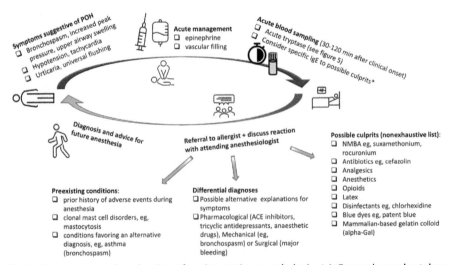

Fig. 2. Description and evaluation of perioperative anaphylaxis. * IgE sample can be taken at time of allergy investigation or be available from preoperative testing (*From* Vitte J, Sabato V, Tacquard C, et al. Use and Interpretation of Acute and Baseline Tryptase in Perioperative Hypersensitivity and Anaphylaxis. J Allergy Clin Immunol Pract. 2021;9(8):2994-3005.)

IgE-mediated reactions to beta-lactams including penicillin, which are the most common culprit antibiotics inducing anaphylactic reactions to antibiotics.[49] One case report involved pruritis, hypotensive syncope, and acutely elevated tryptase following use of B-lactam antibiotics in a patient with elevated basal tryptase.[35,50] Retrospective data have suggested the association of antibiotics and anaphylactic-type reactions in children. In a study consisting of 133 children with various forms of cutaneous mastocytosis, 12 study participants (10%) reported adverse reactions to antibiotics, including 6 to β-lactam antibiotics. Specific details of the reaction severity were not described.[51]

Patients with mastocytosis may be at higher risk for non–IgE-mediated reactions to antibiotics.[31] Those with cutaneous mastocytosis were found to have an increased number of mast cells that express MRGPRX2.[52] This receptor recognizes large cationic molecules such as vancomycin, quinolones, and neuromuscular blockers.[53] In patients with mastocytosis, severe adverse reactions to fluoroquinolones have been reported and are hypothesized to occur via MRGPRX2.[54] Unlike IgE-mediated anaphylaxis, premedication may block or reduce MRGPRX2-related mast cell activation.[55] MRGPRX2-dependant mast cell activation is also a particular concern during perioperative anaphylaxis as described earlier.

Medications that were previously well tolerated may be continued as clinically indicated in patients with a recent diagnosis of mastocytosis. Patients who have exhibited adverse reactions to antibiotics should be evaluated by skin testing and challenge and delabeled if nonreactive. Patients with positive skin test or challenge should benefit from desensitization at times of acute need.

VACCINES

Compared with the general population, patients with mastocytosis are more likely to report adverse reactions following vaccination, but most reactions are mild and are isolated to the skin. Patients with mastocytosis should receive all recommended vaccinations.[30]

Vaccination may trigger mast cell mediator release in children, particularly in those with diffuse cutaneous mastocytosis (DCM). In one study, 44% of children with DCM had evidence of mast cell activation symptoms following vaccination.[56] Corticosteroids, antihistamines, and leukotriene receptor antagonists before vaccination has prevented mast cell activation episodes in some cases.[57]

With respect to messenger RNA (mRNA)-based vaccines, patients seem to have a higher risk of adverse events and anaphylaxis.[58] One respective study examined 323 patients receiving 666 vaccinations.[59] Approximately 6% reported acute adverse events (2% in the general population) and one patient had anaphylaxis. Despite the slight increased rate of adverse reactions in patients with mast cell disorder, mRNA-based vaccines are safe and recommended for patients with mast cell activation disorders.

DRUG ALLERGY IN CHILDREN AND PREGNANT WOMEN

Children with cutaneous mastocytosis are told to avoid antiinflammatory medications, local anesthetics, antibiotics, and RCM. There is little data to support mast cell activation in most of the children with cutaneous or systemic mastocytosis. Children should be evaluated at the time of reactions to drugs, and empirical avoidance of NSAIDs and opioids is not recommended. Pregnancy is not associated with increased mast cell activation, and drugs used during delivery and C-section are well tolerated by most of the patients with cutaneous and systemic mastocytosis.[60]

SUMMARY

"I would like to challenge you with ibuprofen and if you have no reaction, I will remove the label of "Allergy to NSAIDS." You may take aspirin, ibuprofen, and other drugs needed for arthritis. Protocols for skin testing and challenges leading to drug delabeling of mastocytosis patients are needed.

Although some patients with mastocytosis need protection when exposed to NSAIDs, opioids, vaccines, antibiotics, and RCM, better diagnostic tools are needed to assess the populations at risk. Personalized diagnosis should be provided to patients aimed at labeling and delabeling drugs allergies. Patients with mastocytosis should be evaluated for tolerance to drugs before acute situations, particularly children and pregnant women.

New therapies such as tyrosine kinase inhibitors hope to address the number and activation of mast cells and are currently in clinical trials. Whether such medications would improve tolerance of drugs-inducing reactions will need to be addressed.

CLINICS CARE POINTS

- Anaphylaxis to drugs and Hymenoptera should be promptly treated with epinephrine and up to 3 doses may be necessary in patients with high mast cell burden.
- NSAIDs are commonly avoided in patient mastocytosis, and oral challenges should be conducted in both children and adults to assess tolerance.
- Severe reactions to drugs and Hymenoptera venom may be enhanced by the presence of duplicated TPSAB1 genes, and genotyping is recommended for hereditary alpha-tryptasemia.

DISCLOSURE

M.P. Giannetti and M.C. Castells receive funding from Blueprint Medicines and Cogent Biosciences.

REFERENCES

1. Bonadonna P, Scaffidi L. Hymenoptera Anaphylaxis as a Clonal Mast Cell Disorder. Immunol Allergy Clin North Am 2018;38(3). https://doi.org/10.1016/j.iac.2018.04.010.
2. Álvarez-Twose I, Zanotti R, González-De-Olano D, et al. Nonaggressive systemic mastocytosis (SM) without skin lesions associated with insect-induced anaphylaxis shows unique features versus other indolent SM. J Allergy Clin Immunol 2014;133(2). https://doi.org/10.1016/j.jaci.2013.06.020.
3. Bonadonna P, Zanotti R, Müller U. Mastocytosis and insect venom allergy. Curr Opin Allergy Clin Immunol 2010;10(4). https://doi.org/10.1097/ACI.0b013e32833b280c.
4. Neugut AI, Ghatak AT, Miller RL. Anaphylaxis in the United States. Arch Intern Med 2001;161(1). https://doi.org/10.1001/archinte.161.1.15.
5. Panesar SS, Javad S, de Silva D, et al. The epidemiology of anaphylaxis in Europe: A systematic review. Allergy: European Journal of Allergy and Clinical Immunology 2013;68(11). https://doi.org/10.1111/all.12272.
6. Bonadonna P, Perbellini O, Passalacqua G, et al. Clonal mast cell disorders in patients with systemic reactions to Hymenoptera stings and increased serum

tryptase levels. J Allergy Clin Immunol 2009;123(3). https://doi.org/10.1016/j.jaci. 2008.11.018.

7. Brockow K, Jofer C, Behrendt H, et al. Anaphylaxis in patients with mastocytosis: a study on history, clinical features and risk factors in 120 patients. Allergy 2008; 63(2):226–32.

8. González De Olano D, de La Hoz Caballer B, Núñez López R, et al. Prevalence of allergy and anaphylactic symptoms in 210 adult and pediatric patients with mastocytosis in Spain: A study of the Spanish network on mastocytosis (REMA). Clin Exp Allergy 2007;37(10). https://doi.org/10.1111/j.1365-2222.2007.02804.x.

9. Gülen T, Hägglund H, Dahlén B, et al. High prevalence of anaphylaxis in patients with systemic mastocytosis - a single-centre experience. Clin Exp Allergy 2014; 44(1). https://doi.org/10.1111/cea.12225.

10. Oude Elberink J, de Monchy J, Kors J, et al. Fatal anaphylaxis after a yellow jacket sting, despite venom immunotherapy, in two patients with mastocytosis. J Allergy Clin Immunol 1997;99:153–4.

11. Gülen T, Ljung C, Nilsson G, et al. Risk Factor Analysis of Anaphylactic Reactions in Patients With Systemic Mastocytosis. J Allergy Clin Immunol Pract 2017;5(5). https://doi.org/10.1016/j.jaip.2017.02.008.

12. Bonadonna P, Lombardo C, Zanotti R. Mastocytosis and allergic diseases. J Investig Allergol Clin Immunol 2014;24(5).

13. van Anrooij B, van der Veer E, de Monchy JGR, et al. Higher mast cell load decreases the risk of Hymenoptera venom-induced anaphylaxis in patients with mastocytosis. J Allergy Clin Immunol 2013;132(1). https://doi.org/10.1016/j.jaci. 2012.12.1578.

14. Zanotti R, Lombardo C, Passalacqua G, et al. Clonal mast cell disorders in patients with severe Hymenoptera venom allergy and normal serum tryptase levels. J Allergy Clin Immunol 2015;136(1). https://doi.org/10.1016/j.jaci.2014.11.035.

15. Stoevesandt J, Sturm GJ, Bonadonna P, et al. Risk factors and indicators of severe systemic insect sting reactions. Allergy 2020;75(3). https://doi.org/10.1111/all.13945.

16. Bonifazi F, Jutel M, Biló BM, et al. Prevention and treatment of hymenoptera venom allergy: Guidelines for clinical practice. Allergy 2005;60(12). https://doi. org/10.1111/j.1398-9995.2005.00960.x.

17. Kleine-Tebbe J, Matricardi PM, Hamilton RG. Allergy Work-Up Including Component-Resolved Diagnosis: How to Make Allergen-Specific Immunotherapy More Specific. Immunol Allergy Clin North Am 2016;36(1). https://doi.org/10. 1016/j.iac.2015.08.012.

18. González-de-Olano D, Padial-Vilchez MA, Núñez-Acevedo B, et al. Usefulness of omalizumab and sting challenge test in hymenoptera venom allergy and mastocytosis. J Investig Allergol Clin Immunol 2019;29(4). https://doi.org/10.18176/jiaci.0395.

19. González-De-Olano D, Álvarez-Twose I, Vega A, et al. Venom immunotherapy in patients with mastocytosis and hymenoptera venom anaphylaxis. Immunotherapy 2011;3(5). https://doi.org/10.2217/imt.11.44.

20. Romantowski J, Gorska A, Lange M, et al. How to diagnose mast cell activation syndrome: Practical considerations. Pol Arch Intern Med 2020;130(4). https://doi. org/10.20452/pamw.15212.

21. Jarkvist J, Salehi C, Akin C, et al. Venom immunotherapy in patients with clonal mast cell disorders: IgG4 correlates with protection. Allergy 2020;75(1). https:// doi.org/10.1111/all.13980.

22. Giannetti M, Silver J, Hufdhi R, et al. One-day ultrarush desensitization for Hymenoptera venom anaphylaxis in patients with and without mast cell disorders with adjuvant omalizumab. J Allergy Clin Immunol Pract 2020;8(4). https://doi.org/10.1016/j.jaip.2019.10.022.

23. Rama TA, Morgado JM, Henriques A, et al. Mastocytosis presenting with mast cell-mediator release-associated symptoms elicited by cyclo oxygenase inhibitors: prevalence, clinical, and laboratory features. Clin Transl Allergy 2022;12(3). https://doi.org/10.1002/clt2.12132.

24. Butterfield JH. Survey of aspirin administration in systemic mastocytosis. Prostaglandins Other Lipid Mediat 2009;88(3–4):122–4. https://doi.org/10.1016/j.prostaglandins.2009.01.001.

25. Aun MV, Blanca M, Garro LS, et al. Nonsteroidal anti-inflammatory drugs are major causes of drug-induced anaphylaxis. J Allergy Clin Immunol Pract 2014;2(4):414–20.

26. Bonadonna P, Pagani M, Aberer W, et al. Drug hypersensitivity in clonal mast cell disorders: ENDA/EAACI position paper. Allergy 2015;70(7):755–63.

27. Schwartz LB, Metcalfe DD, Miller JS, et al. Tryptase levels as an indicator of mast-cell activation in systemic anaphylaxis and mastocytosis. N Engl J Med 1987;316:1622–6.

28. Butterfield JH, Kao PC, Klee GG, et al. Aspirin Idiosyncrasy in systemic mast cell disease: a new look at mediator release during aspirin desensitization. Mayo Clin Proc 1995;70:481–7.

29. Pfeffer I, Fischer J, Biedermann T. Acetylsalicylsäure-abhängige anaphylaxie auf karotte bei mastozytose. JDDG 2011;9(3):230–1.

30. Carter MC, Metcalfe DD, Matito A, et al. Adverse reactions to drugs and biologics in patients with clonal mast cell disorders: A Work Group Report of the Mast Cells Disorder Committee, American Academy of Allergy, Asthma & Immunology. J Allergy Clin Immunol 2019;143(3):880–93.

31. Butterfield JH, Weiler CR. Prevention of mast cell activation disorder-associated clinical sequelae of excessive prostaglandin D2 production. Int Arch Allergy Immunol 2008;147(4):338–43.

32. Roberts L, Fields J, Oates J. Mastocytosis without urticaria pigmentosa: a frequently unrecognized cause of recurrent syncope. Trans Assoc Am Physicians 1982;95:36–41.

33. Cochran ST, Bomyea K, Sayre JW. Trends in adverse events after IV Administration of contrast media A.; 2001. www.ajronline.org.

34. Álvarez-Twose I, González de Olano D, Sánchez-Muñoz L, et al. Clinical, biological, and molecular characteristics of clonal mast cell disorders presenting with systemic mast cell activation symptoms. J Allergy Clin Immunol 2010;125(6). https://doi.org/10.1016/j.jaci.2010.02.019.

35. Bonadonna P, Lombardo C. Drug allergy in mastocytosis. Immunol Allergy Clin North Am 2014;34(2):397–405.

36. Brockow K, Romano A, Aberer W, et al. Skin testing in patients with hypersensitivity reactions to iodinated contrast media - A European multicenter study. Allergy 2009;64(2):234–41.

37. Weingarten T, Volcheck G, Sprung J. Anaphylactoid reaction to intravenous contrast in patient with systemic mastocytosis. Anaesth Intensive Care 2009;37:646–9.

38. Isabwe GAC, Garcia Neuer M, de las Vecillas Sanchez L, et al. Hypersensitivity reactions to therapeutic monoclonal antibodies: Phenotypes and endotypes. J Allergy Clin Immunol 2018;142(1):159–70.e2.

39. Bernaola M, Hamadi SA, Lynch DM, et al. Successful administration of omalizumab by desensitization protocol following systemic reactions in 12 patients. J Allergy Clin Immunol Pract 2021;9(6):2505–8.
40. Blunk JA, Schmelz M, Zeck S, et al. Opioid-Induced Mast Cell Activation and Vascular Responses Is Not Mediated by μ-Opioid Receptors: An In Vivo Microdialysis Study in Human Skin. Anesth Analg 2004;98(2):364–70.
41. Rosow C, Philbin D, Deegan CR, et al. Hemodynamics and histamine release during induction with sufentanil or fentanyl. Anesthesiology 1984;60:489–91.
42. Mertes PM, Alla F, Tréchot P, et al. Anaphylaxis during anesthesia in France: An 8-year national survey. J Allergy Clin Immunol 2011;128(2):366–73.
43. Matito A, Morgado JM, Sánchez-López P, et al. Management of Anesthesia in Adult and Pediatric Mastocytosis: A Study of the Spanish Network on Mastocytosis (REMA) Based on 726 Anesthetic Procedures. Int Arch Allergy Immunol 2015; 167(1):47–56.
44. Hermans MAW, Arends NJT, Gerth van Wijk R, et al. Management around invasive procedures in mastocytosis: An update. Ann Allergy Asthma Immunol 2017;119(4):304–9.
45. Stellato C, Casolaro V, Ciccarelli A, et al. General ANAESTHETICS INDUCE ONLY HISTAMINE RELEASE SELECTIVELY FROM HUMAN MAST CELLS. Vol 67.; 1991.
46. Stellato C, de Paulis A, Cirillo R, et al. Heterogeneity of human mast cells and basophils in response to muscle relaxants. Anesthesiology 1991;74:1078–86.
47. Roy S, Chompunud Na Ayudhya C, Thapaliya M, et al. Multifaceted MRGPRX2: New insight into the role of mast cells in health and disease. J Allergy Clin Immunol 2021;148(2):293–308.
48. Broesby-Olsen S, Farkas DK, Vestergaard H, et al. Risk of solid cancer, cardiovascular disease, anaphylaxis, osteoporosis and fractures in patients with systemic mastocytosis: A nationwide population-based study. Am J Hematol 2016; 91(11):1069–75.
49. Castells M, Khan DA, Phillips EJ. Penicillin Allergy. In: Longo DL, editor. N Engl J Med 2019;381(24):2338–51.
50. Alonso Díaz De Durana MD, Fernández-Rivas M, Casas ML, et al. Anaphylaxis during negative penicillin skin prick testing confirmed by elevated serum tryptase. Allergy: European Journal of Allergy and Clinical Immunology 2003; 58(2):159.
51. Schena D, Galvan A, Tessari G, et al. Clinical features and course of cutaneous mastocytosis in 133 children. Br J Dermatol 2016;174(2):411–3.
52. Deepak V, Komarow HD, Alblaihess AA, et al. Expression of MRGPRX2 in skin mast cells of patients with maculopapular cutaneous mastocytosis. J Allergy Clin Immunol Pract 2021;9(10):3841–3.e1.
53. McNeil BD, Pundir P, Meeker S, et al. Identification of a mast-cell-specific receptor crucial for pseudo-allergic drug reactions. Nature 2015;519(7542):237–41.
54. Giavina-Bianchi P, Gonçalves DG, Zanandréa A, et al. Anaphylaxis to quinolones in mastocytosis: Hypothesis on the mechanism. J Allergy Clin Immunol Pract 2019;7(6):2089–90.
55. Renz CL, Laroche D, Thurn JD, et al. Tryptase Levels Are Not Increased during Vancomycin-induced Anaphylactoid Reactions. Anesthesiology 1998;89(3):620–5.
56. Alvarez-Twose I, Vañó-Galván S, Sánchez-Muñoz L, et al. Increased serum baseline tryptase levels and extensive skin involvement are predictors for the severity of mast cell activation episodes in children with mastocytosis. Allergy 2012;67(6): 813–21.

57. Bankova LG, Walter JE, Iyengar SR, et al. Generalized Bullous Eruption after Routine Vaccination in a Child with Diffuse Cutaneous Mastocytosis. J Allergy Clin Immunol Pract 2013;1(1):94–6.

58. Bonadonna P, Brockow K, Niedoszytko M, et al. COVID-19 Vaccination in Mastocytosis: Recommendations of the European Competence Network on Mastocytosis (ECNM) and American Initiative in Mast Cell Diseases (AIM). J Allergy Clin Immunol Pract 2021;9(6):2139–44.

59. Giannetti MP, Olivieri F, Godwin G, et al. Outcomes of COVID-19 vaccination in 323 patients with clonal and non-clonal mast cell activation disorders. Allergy 2022. https://doi.org/10.1111/all.15476.

60. Matito A, Álvarez-Twose I, Morgado JM, et al. Clinical impact of pregnancy in mastocytosis: A study of the Spanish network on mastocytosis (REMA) in 45 cases. Int Arch Allergy Immunol 2011;156(1):104–11.

Gastrointestinal Disease in Mastocytosis

Matthew J. Hamilton, MD

KEYWORDS

- Mastocytosis • Gastrointestinal • Endoscopy • Abdominal pain • Diarrhea • Peptic
- Cromolyn

KEY POINTS

- Gastrointestinal symptoms in patients with systemic mastocytosis (SM) are prominent and contribute to significant morbidity.
- In indolent SM, the gastrointestinal symptoms are mainly due to mast cell mediator release but may be due to non–mast cell factors that can be deciphered during the diagnostic workup.
- Patients with advanced SM may experience signs and symptoms of gastrointestinal and hepatic dysfunction owing to the massive infiltration of clonal mast cells in the tissues.
- Gastrointestinal symptoms in SM are treatable with a combination of mast cell–directed therapies, mediations to treat specific symptoms, and dietary modification.

INTRODUCTION

It has long been appreciated that gastrointestinal (GI) symptoms are prominent in patients with systemic mastocytosis (SM). Studies that have evaluated the frequency of symptoms among patients with SM consistently show the GI organ system to be among the most affected.[1–4] Furthermore, these symptoms, which include heartburn and reflux, nausea, abdominal bloat, abdominal cramping, and loose stools, are a significant source of morbidity for patients.

Despite the impact of these symptoms in SM, there is a paucity of published literature regarding the pathogenesis of GI manifestations of the disease. From a diagnostic standpoint, the pathologic features of SM in the intestine have only recently been appreciated, and questions remain as to how these findings may be used to guide treatment. In this article, the GI symptoms commonly observed in SM will be reviewed with regards to diagnostic considerations and management.

Mastocytosis Center, Brigham and Women's Hospital, Crohn's and Colitis Center, Harvard Medical School, 850 Boylston Street, Chestnut Hill, MA 02467, USA
E-mail address: mjhamilton@bwh.harvard.edu

Immunol Allergy Clin N Am 43 (2023) 711–722
https://doi.org/10.1016/j.iac.2023.04.005
0889-8561/23/© 2023 Elsevier Inc. All rights reserved.
immunology.theclinics.com

BACKGROUND

Mast cells are thought to play important roles in the intestine with regards to pathogen defense, intestinal barrier function, and intestinal homeostasis among other key roles.[5] In pathologic conditions, mast cells may contribute to increased intestinal permeability, secretion of solutes and fluid into the intestinal lumen, inflammation propagation, pain perception, and changes in intestinal motility.[6] SM is characterized by an influx of clonal mast cells into the tissues, including the GI tract. In order to understand what may be driving GI symptoms in SM, it is important to distinguish between different causes among the different SM types.

Much of this article focuses on the GI symptoms and manifestations observed in patients with indolent disease whereby symptoms are largely driven by mast cell activation and potentially other causes related to the physiology of mast cell mediator release in the tissues.[3,7] In the more advanced forms of SM, the cause of intestinal symptoms is due in part to mast cell mediator release but also to the effect of the significant mast cell burden at the absorptive surface of the intestine. This manifestation leads to interference of water and solute transport and may result in diarrhea and potentially malabsorption of nutrients. A third category of GI symptoms in patients with SM is related to non–mast cell–related factors, such as medication side effects or comorbid diseases that also manifest with GI symptoms.

The description of the manifestations of SM are therefore broken down by symptom type for indolent SM and advanced SM. The diagnostic tests that are performed to clarify symptom cause are described as well as personalized treatments.

GASTROINTESTINAL MANIFESTATIONS OF INDOLENT SYSTEMIC MASTOCYTOSIS
Peptic-Specific Symptoms

Patients with SM commonly present with symptoms attributed to increased gastric acid production[8] (**Table 1**). The release of histamine from tissue resident mast cells in the stomach may stimulate acid production by binding to histamine 2 receptors (H2R) in the acid-producing parietal cells. Peptic symptoms, which include heartburn and acid reflux, are among the more common GI symptoms experienced by patients with SM.

Peptic disease may manifest with reflux esophagitis, which could cause more persistent symptoms of heartburn, noncardiac chest pain, and swallowing difficulties, such as solid food dysphagia. Patients may also experience gastritis with dyspepsia symptoms, including nausea and epigastric pain. On endoscopy, patients may have evidence of ulcer disease in the gastric antrum and pylorus. Symptoms may include persistent pain felt in the epigastric area.

In addition, patients may present with GI bleeding owing to an exposed blood vessel in the ulcer bed or signs and symptoms of gastric outlet obstruction owing to the local

Table 1	
Gastrointestinal symptom presentation in systemic mastocytosis	
Mast cell mediator symptoms	Nausea Abdominal cramping Loose stools
Mastocytosis-specific symptoms	Peptic: heartburn or reflux Chronic diarrhea with malabsorption (advanced)
Nonspecific symptoms	Vomiting Abdominal distension Constipation

inflammatory effect of the ulcer. Patients with SM may also have peptic ulcer disease in the duodenum and will present in a similar way, although there may be subtle differences in the characterization of symptoms. The pain attributed to duodenal ulcers is often worse after eating owing to stimulation of acid production. SM is in the differential diagnosis for a patient who presents with multiple ulcers in the various segments of the duodenum.

Upper Gastrointestinal Tract Symptoms Related to Mast Cell Mediator Release

Patients with indolent SM may experience symptoms involving the upper GI tract when exposed to various triggers that result in mast cell mediator release. Although it is not known if there are any specific mediators that drive particular GI symptoms, prostaglandins, histamines, and tryptase have all been implicated owing to their effects on the GI tract.

Symptoms that are specific to mast cell mediator release include nausea and associated abdominal cramp feelings (see **Table 1**). This often occurs within minutes of an ingested meal or any other trigger for mast cell activation symptoms. The duration of the symptoms is variable and may be related to factors such as the amount of time of exposure to the trigger (eg, 6–12 hours for a food substance). GI symptoms that are related to mast cell mediator release are responsive to treatments with mast cell medicator blocking medications (see later discussion in the treatment section).[9]

Nausea and more rarely vomiting may occur even in the absence of trigger owing to other factors. Nausea in general is a nonspecific symptom with many causes, including food intolerance, gastric-emptying delay, other forms of gastritis, or even non-GI causes, such as central neurologic disorders.

Lower Intestinal Symptoms Related to Mast Cell Mediator Release

"Diarrhea" is frequently listed as a symptom of SM, but this is a nonspecific term and does not account for the range in bowel movement symptoms patients experience nor the many potential causes (see **Table 1**). In well-controlled indolent SM, patients typically have formed and daily bowel movements. Symptomatic patients may experience onset of loose stools with a trigger within hours, and the change in bowel movement pattern may last up to days. Stools are often solid at first but become more loose and even watery with increased stool frequency and urgency. Blood and mucous in the stool are not typically seen, and the stools typically begin to form again once the effect of the trigger has passed. Patients may even describe constipation for a period of time after a mast cell activation event. Patients with indolent SM do not typically experience chronic, persistent loose stools and should be investigated for other causes if this exists.

Although there are no known GI conditions that are more commonly associated with SM, patients may have comorbid intestinal inflammatory conditions, such as inflammatory bowel disease, celiac disease, or microscopic colitis. Food intolerance and medication side effects are commonly observed in this patient population and should also be considered with more chronic and continuous loose stools. Constipation may be seen in patients with well-controlled SM who are not having frequent mast cell activation reactions. This symptom may be due to underlying idiopathic constipation, medication side effects (eg, antihistamines, antidepressants, pain medications), or dietary factors, such as inadequate fiber intake.

A symptom that is commonly associated with onset of loose stools is abdominal cramping. This may be felt anywhere in the abdomen but is described most often as occurring in the mid area around the umbilicus. Patients also often describe a sensation of "bloat" whereby they feel as though their abdomen is more protuberant. True abdominal distension may also be experienced, especially if they have baseline constipation. Typically, the abdominal cramps and bloat sensation will start within minutes to hours after the trigger and before the bowel movements become loose and ultimately improve once the bowel movements begin to form again.

Patients with indolent SM may experience abdominal pain symptoms in various locations even in the absence of mast cell activation events and for unknown reasons. However, patients with well-controlled SM do not have frequent abdominal pain, and providers should have a low threshold in these cases to investigate for other potential causes of pain, such as organ-specific disease (eg, biliary and pancreas), constipation, malignancy, and inflammatory conditions.

Diagnostic Considerations for Gastrointestinal Symptoms in Indolent Systemic Mastocytosis

Patients with indolent SM who are experiencing typical GI symptoms of mast cell activation (onset of heartburn and nausea followed by abdominal cramping and loose stools after a trigger), and which are often associated with symptoms in other organ systems, such as pruritis and flushing, are tested for elevations of mast cell mediators, including serum tryptase and metabolites of histamine, prostaglandin, and leukotriene in the urine. The levels are then compared with a baseline set of laboratory values. There are no other laboratory, endoscopic, or radiographic tests that can be used to correlate GI symptoms with mast cell activation (**Box 1**).

These additional tests in the symptomatic patient with SM are often done to rule out other conditions. When persistent upper abdominal pain, early satiety, dysphagia, evidence of GI bleeding, or weight loss is present, cross-sectional abdominal imaging with computed tomography or MRI and upper endoscopy are performed.

Upper endoscopy is used to evaluate the esophagus, stomach, and duodenum portion of the small intestine. This test is sensitive to detect anatomical changes, such as strictures and tumors. The endoscopist will be able to assess for the presence and extent of peptic ulcer disease and whether there are complications, such as stigmata of bleeding or intestinal obstruction. Segmental biopsies are often performed whereby the pathologist can then assess for underlying inflammatory conditions (eg, celiac, eosinophilic disorders), infection (*Helicobacter pylori*), autoimmune conditions (gastritis), or malignancy or premalignant conditions (eg, lymphoma, adenocarcinoma).

Box 1
Systemic mastocytosis clinical and laboratory evaluation specific to gastrointestinal

Clinical evaluation
- History taking and evaluation of symptoms
- Documentation of triggers
- Complete abdominal examination with assessment of organomegaly (liver and spleen)
- Evaluation for signs of malabsorption (eg, ascites)

Medical and laboratory tests
- CBC with differential
- Liver function tests, including serum albumin, and serum alkaline phosphatase
- Laboratory tests that indicate malabsorption, including iron studies, folate, B12, INR
- Endoscopy and colonoscopy with biopsies
  - CD117, CD25
- Cross-sectional imaging with abdominal CT or MRI

Abbreviations: CBC, complete blood count; CT, computed tomography; INR, international normalized ratio.

When lower GI symptoms are prominent, cross-sectional imaging is helpful to evaluate acute onset or chronic abdominal pain symptoms. Colonoscopy with biopsy is helpful to assess for inflammatory conditions, including inflammatory bowel disease including microscopic colitis, diverticular disease, and malignancy.

In the patient with SM with persistent GI symptoms, not improved with mast cell medications and with no other explanation after completion of the standard testing, other tests are available to evaluate symptoms. Manometry and gastric-emptying tests can assess for primary or secondary GI motility disorders, and breath tests can assess for specific food intolerances, such as lactose and fructose. A breath test may also be done to assess for small intestinal bacterial overgrowth, which may be seen in someone with significant impairment of GI motility or history of intestinal resection surgery. There are no specific intestinal microbial abnormalities that have been identified in patients with SM nor are there mainstream clinical tests to assess for microbial imbalances that may or may not exist in this population.

Specific Gastrointestinal Diagnostic Testing in Patients with Indolent Systemic Mastocytosis

In patients with SM who have prominent GI symptoms as part of their mast cell activation symptomology or more persistent symptoms of abdominal pain and loose stools, endoscopy and colonoscopy with intestinal biopsy can be used to determine the extent of clonal mast cell involvement of the intestine (**Fig. 1**; see **Box 1**).

Biopsies obtained at endoscopy typically include the mucosal layer and occasionally the submucosa. In normal intestine, mast cells are dispersed throughout the lamina propria portion of the mucosa and are typically not seen at the surface epithelium or epithelial crypts. Normal mast cells in the intestine are round cells with an ovoid nucleus and clear cytoplasm. They have also been described as irregularly shaped with spindle formation.[10]

The number of mast cells observed per high-power field varies by region of the intestine (stomach vs colon) but is typically 15 to 25 mast cells per high-power field of view. The clinical utility of quantifying mast cells on intestinal biopsies has not been shown to be useful to distinguish between irritable bowel syndrome and mast cell activation syndrome, although it could be helpful to a pathologist who is considering SM

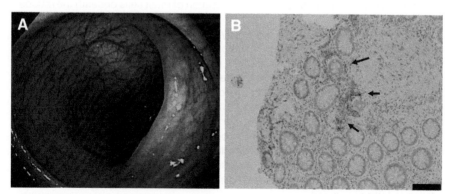

Fig. 1. Colonoscopy and histopathology in indolent SM. The appearance of the colon during colonoscopy can be normal (*A*), although nonspecific findings have been reported, such as nodules and erythematous patches. Random and targeted biopsies taken throughout the colon may reveal characteristic aggregates of greater than 15 mast cells and that stain for CD25 (*B*; arrows). 40x magnification, CD25 stain.

when the number of mast cells per high-power field is elevated. In a retrospective study that described the intestinal features of 24 cases of SM, the mean number of mast cells across 5 high-power fields was 125 (range, 42–278) compared with 19 (7–39) in a control population.[11]

The clonal mast cells in the intestine diagnostic of SM have similar characteristics of those observed in the bone marrow that have been well documented and define the major criterion for a diagnosis of SM. In cases of indolent SM, clonal mast cells in the intestinal mucosa are found in aggregates of 15 or more[11,12] and stain positively for the cell surface marker CD25 with immunohistochemistry. In indolent disease, clonal mast cells may also be found in "sheets" or a "bandlike" distribution beneath the mucosal layer. This finding is more commonly observed as the mast cell burden increases in advanced mastocytosis and where there may be diffuse and compact infiltration of mast cells in the lamia propria. Prominent eosinophilia has also been observed in up to 50% of SM cases and may be another clue to a pathologist to suspect SM.[3,11,12]

The degree of GI symptoms of mast cell activation has not been shown to correlate with the degree of clonal mast cell burden in the intestine in indolent disease.[3] Patients with prominent upper GI symptoms may not have a significant burden of clonal mast cells in the stomach, and those with a high burden of clonal mast cells in the stomach do not necessarily have a lot of nausea and abdominal cramping.

In general, the highest-yield location to identify clonal mast cells in the intestine is the colon, followed by the small intestine (ileum and duodenum), followed by the stomach.[11] The presence of clonal mucosal intestinal mast cells has not been extensively studied in the esophagus or mid small intestine nor deeper layers of the intestine, including the submucosa and muscle layer.

Endoscopic features of indolent SM may include nodules and polyps, although this may be due to the fact that endoscopists typically biopsy or remove polyps that are then available for review by the pathology department. In order to detect features of SM in the intestine, multiple random biopsies are taken in each intestinal segment. Endoscopists do not typically take biopsies in patients who do not have chronic GI symptoms and who have normal-appearing colons, and so, the decision to take random biopsies is made before the procedure.

The endoscopic features of patients with advanced SM include a congested appearance likely owing to the significant infiltration of mast cells beneath the mucosal surface (**Fig. 2**).

Endoscopy with biopsies is diagnostically useful in a patient with suspected SM in order to satisfy the diagnostic criteria. Although the bone marrow biopsy is the standard of care to make the diagnosis of SM, a patient with prominent GI symptoms may have endoscopy and colonoscopy with intestinal segmental biopsies that ultimately satisfy the major criterion for SM with the identification of aggregates of 15 or more mast cells and minor criteria including CD25+ mast cells and abnormally spindle-shaped mast cells. If a patient satisfies the diagnostic criteria on intestinal biopsies, it is still recommended that they undergo bone marrow biopsy to assess for other hematologic conditions for final disease classification.

Endoscopy and colonoscopy with biopsies are also important in the patient with advanced SM with new or persistent GI symptoms especially with diarrhea and are detailed in later discussion.

Therapeutic Approach to Gastrointestinal Symptoms in Systemic Mastocytosis

A therapy plan can be devised for a patient with SM once the symptoms have been reviewed and cataloged (**Table 2**). Treatment considerations are tailored to the

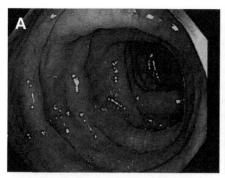
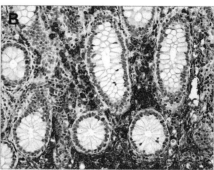

Fig. 2. Colonoscopy and histopathology in advanced SM. The colon may have a congested appearance with patchy erythema (*A*). Random biopsies reveal densely packed infiltrates of clonal mast cells throughout the lamina propria portion of the mucosa (*B*; tryptase stain) and underneath the epithelial surface layer. 40x magnification, CD25 stain.

symptoms of mast cell activation, SM-specific treatments, and other disorders or factors causing GI symptoms.

In patients with mast cell activation-type symptoms, the standard step-up approach is used.[13] Although the efficacy of this standard treatment approach has not been specifically analyzed in SM, results of a small retrospective study of patients with mast cell activation syndrome showed that the GI symptoms attributed to mast cell activation were readily treated. Both histamine 1 receptor antagonist and H2R antagonists can be used alone or in combination and at the lowest dosage that successfully treats symptoms.[14] Specific to GI symptoms, the H2R antihistamines have the added benefit of serving as an antacid, which may be beneficial for those with peptic-type symptoms of heartburn, reflux, and nausea.

The mast cell stabilizer oral sodium cromolyn may be added to antihistamines or used first line to treat the GI symptoms of SM.[15] Although the mechanism of action of oral cromolyn to treat systemic symptoms is not fully known, it is possible that orally ingested and poorly absorbed cromolyn works optimally in the GI tract. This is typically taken in liquid form at doses of 600 to 800 mg a day, although there are no standard doses that have been approved for cromolyn, and the dose can be titrated to effect. Side effects of cromolyn are primarily GI, and nausea and increased abdominal cramping are commonly observed. For maximal treatment response, it is recommended that cromolyn be taken in divided doses 3 to 4 times a day and on an empty stomach.

Table 2
Treatment options for systemic mastocytosis

	ISM and AdvSM	AdvSM Only
Mast cell mediator symptoms	Antihistamines, oral cromolyn sodium	
SM-specific medications	PPI	Budesonide, corticosteroids
GI-specific symptoms	Ondansetron: nausea Loperamide: antidiarrheal Short-acting anticholinergics (eg, hyoscyamine): abdominal cramping Laxatives: constipation	

Abbreviations: AdvSM, advanced systemic mastocytosis; ISM, indolent systemic mastocytosis.

In addition to histamine, other mast cell mediators have been implicated in the genesis of GI symptoms, and additional medications that block mediators may be added depending on the treatment response to antihistamines and oral cromolyn. These may include leukotriene blockers (eg, montelukast) and aspirin to block prostaglandin production. However, aspirin should be used with caution in a patient population who is already at increased risk of peptic ulcer disease. Doses of aspirin up to 325 mg daily are likely to be safe and especially if combined with a proton-pump inhibitor antacid (PPI), although this treatment has not been studied in SM.

The GI symptoms of mast cell activation in patients with SM are well treated with the standard treatment approach outlined above. In patients with refractory symptoms, treatment with small molecule tyrosine kinase inhibitors that selectively inhibit activation-loop mutants of KIT, including D816V, have been shown to reduce GI symptoms in patients with advanced disease.[16,17] It is likely that the reduction of symptoms observed with this type of treatment is due to reduction in mast cell burden. These treatments are being evaluated for the treatment of indolent disease, and it remains to be seen whether symptoms of mast cell mediator release will be reduced in these patients without a significant mast cell burden. In advanced disease, the greatest GI symptom reduction was with avapritinib, as opposed to midostaurin, which may have GI side effects, including nausea and vomiting.[16]

In addition to mast cell–specific treatments, there are symptom-directed medical therapies for patients with ongoing GI symptoms. The treatment approach is similar to those with irritable bowel syndrome and includes medications directed at pain (eg, tricyclic antidepressants [TCAs]), diarrhea (eg, imodium), nausea (ondansetron), and fiber supplementation to form the stool.[18]

For the peptic manifestations of SM, including heartburn and acid reflux symptoms, and gastric or duodenal ulcer prevention or treatment, PPI antacids may be used. These are considered safe for short-term use and are well tolerated. Although the incidence of peptic ulcer disease in patients with SM has not been studied over time, it is anticipated that PPI use has contributed to a reduction in morbidity from peptic ulcer disease.

Particular attention to diet is important in all patients with GI symptoms, including those with SM. Food intolerances, including lactose, gluten/wheat, and food additives and preservatives, are common in patients with SM and were reported to occur in 40% to 50% of patients in one survey-based study.[19] Careful restriction can improve symptoms of food intolerance that include nausea, abdominal bloat, and loose stools after ingestion of the food substance. Certain foods may be specific triggers for mast cell mediator release symptoms, and so restriction of these foods is also beneficial. In order to ensure that patients are consuming a well-rounded diet sufficient in protein, calories, and nutrients, a consult with a dietician is often necessary.

Gastrointestinal Manifestations of Advanced Systemic Mastocytosis Including Diagnosis and Treatment

Patients with advanced SM are defined as meeting the standard criteria for SM and additionally displaying at least one "C" finding.[20] One of these findings is malabsorption and weight loss owing to the mast cell burden in the intestine. Patients with malabsorption typically report greasy-type, loose stools that may float and are foul-smelling. Weight loss and micronutrient (eg, iron, folate, vitamin K) and macronutrient (protein) deficiencies are common. Patients may experience weight loss and third-spacing of fluids owing to protein-losing enteropathy. Malabsorption is often a clinical diagnosis in patients with advanced SM and may be confirmed with laboratory testing of serum albumin and prealbumin and various micronutrients. Endoscopy and colonoscopy with biopsy are considered in patients with refractory symptoms or with additional symptoms, such as GI bleeding. The endoscopic and histologic features of advanced SM were described previously.

The treatment of patients with advanced SM who have symptoms owing to the massive mast cell infiltration, including diarrhea and weight loss, are largely directed at reducing the mast cell burden. If chronic GI symptoms continue, corticosteroids have anecdotally been used to reduce mast cell burden in the intestine and reduce symptoms. Budesonide is a type of steroid with very little systemic absorption (<5%) and is released into the distal small intestine and colon. Although it has not formerly been studied in SM, one small study documented treatment effect in a population of patients with "mastocytic enterocolitis" who had increased GI symptoms in association with elevated numbers of mast cells in the colon.[21]

In addition to clonal mast cell infiltration in the intestine, patients with SM may have evidence of liver involvement. A "B" finding that may suggest smoldering SM is the presence of hepatomegaly without impairment in liver function or splenomegaly. The presence of one "C" finding to suggest advanced SM is the presence of palpable hepatomegaly with impairment of liver function, ascites, or portal hypertension.[20]

In the largest published series of patients with SM that assessed hepatic involvement, about half of the 41 patients had liver blood test abnormalities and a quarter had hepatomegaly.[22] The extent of liver involvement increased with severity of mastocytosis and was rarely seen in indolent disease and most commonly seen in advanced SM. Histologic abnormalities included infiltration with fibrosis adjacent to the portal tracts and sinusoids and to a lesser degree the liver parenchyma. Cirrhosis was not observed, and so, the clinical finding of hepatomegaly and ascites in patients with advanced SM is likely due to the burden of infiltrating mast cells at the portal areas causing portal hypertension. Hepatic synthetic dysfunction is rarely seen in patients with SM.

DISCUSSION, INCLUDING CONTROVERSIES

It remains unknown whether there are cases of isolated mastocytosis in the intestine that have clinical significance. A study described 16 patients who were incidentally found to have the pathologic features of mastocytosis in the intestine but who did not have any other clinical features to suggest SM and who in some cases had negative bone marrow investigations.[23] Although several of these patients had follow-up evaluations, a larger registry of patients with long-term data will be necessary to determine whether any of these patients develop SM with positive bone marrow evaluations consistent with the diagnosis and symptoms and other manifestations of SM.

Although not published, CD25+ mast cells have been observed in intestinal biopsies in patients with symptoms of mast cell activation but who do not meet other criteria to suggest SM. It is not known if this finding could represent a feature of monoclonal mast cell activation syndrome[24] or is a precursor to SM. Larger registries of patients and longitudinal data are needed to determine the significance of this finding.

There are currently no guidelines for what represents a normal number of mast cells in the intestine. In syndromes with prominent GI symptoms, such as irritable bowel syndrome[25] and mast cell activation syndrome,[10] there is a range in the number of intestinal mast cells, although the mean number is close to what is observed in people without a mast cell disorder or GI symptoms. Although the mean numbers of mast cells are increased in the intestine in patients with SM and may be the first clue to this diagnosis, the pathognomonic finding remains the presence of aggregates or sheets of greater than 15 mast cells that stain positively for CD25. Intestinal mast cells in patients with hereditary alpha-tryptasemia (HaT) were also observed in aggregates but composed of fewer than 15 mast cells.[10]

It is not always clear what drives GI symptoms in patients with SM. In those who have significant mast cell mediator release–type symptoms with concurrent flushing and airway symptoms, trials of medications to target mast cell mediators may be therapeutic as well as diagnostic to see if these specific symptoms improve. In the future, treatment with clonal mast cell–reducing therapies, such as the tyrosine kinase inhibitors, may provide insight into whether the population of clonal mast cells in the intestine in indolent disease has a significant impact on GI symptoms or whether this treatment effect is simply a systemic effect on mast cell activation. The finding of clonal mast cells in the intestine does not always correlate with GI symptoms.[3]

Patients with certain mast cell disorders, including mast cell activation syndrome and HaT, have been reported in one study to be associated with autonomic dysfunction and small fiber neuropathy in patients with neurologic type symptoms.[26] Although the prevalence of these associated conditions has not been studied in SM, it is possible that abdominal pain and underlying intestinal motility defects may be caused by pathogenic mast cell–nerve fiber interactions innervating the intestine.[25,27] Comprehensive autonomic testing in patients with SM with and without postural and neuropathy symptoms would help to answer this question.

Although mast cells have been implicated in colorectal cancer pathogenesis and precancerous colon polyp formation,[28] there are no large series that show an increased incidence of colon cancer or adenoma polyps in patients with SM, and accordingly, there are no specific cancer screening guidelines. An association between SM and other intestinal inflammatory conditions, such as celiac disease, inflammatory bowel disease, and eosinophilic disorders, has not been established, although these conditions may coexist with SM and should be considered in those with refractory GI symptoms.

SUMMARY

The GI symptoms experienced by patients with SM are common and contribute to the significant morbidity patients experience. The cause is frequently a manifestation of mast cell mediator release upon exposure to a trigger, but there are many other factors that may be indirectly or not related to SM that cause symptoms. A thorough workup that includes radiology and endoscopy with intestinal biopsies may help in the diagnostic evaluation and assist with management when symptoms persist. Treatment that includes therapies directed at mast cells and mast cell mediators, GI symptom–directed therapies, and dietary modifications is effective. Although it is clear that GI manifestations in patients with advanced disease are due to the massive infiltration of clonal mast cells that effect function, future studies are necessary to determine what mechanisms may contribute to GI signs and symptoms in indolent disease.

CLINICS CARE POINTS

- When evaluating a patient with systemic mastocytosis and gastrointestinal symptoms, determine which of the symptoms are related to mast cell activation and which may be due to other causes. Treatment, including mast cell–directed therapies and symptom-based medications, is titrated accordingly.

- During the diagnostic workup for a patient suspected of systemic mastocytosis with gastrointestinal symptoms, consider endoscopy and colonoscopy with random biopsies and staining to assess for the presence and extent of the clonal mast cells.

- If a patient with systemic mastocytosis continues to have gastrointestinal symptoms despite adequate mast cell–directed therapies, evaluate for comorbid conditions, such as primary gastrointestinal disorders and medication and food intolerances.
- Remember that dietary factors are a significant driver of gastrointestinal symptoms in patients with systemic mastocytosis, and careful review of allergies and intolerances is an integral part of the treatment plan along with ensuring that the patient is consuming a well-balanced diet.

CONFLICT OF INTEREST

There are no conflicts of interest to disclose that are relevant to the content in this article.

REFERENCES

1. van Anrooij B, Kluin-Nelemans JC, Safy M, et al. Patient-reported disease-specific quality-of-life and symptom severity in systemic mastocytosis. Allergy: European Journal of Allergy and Clinical Immunology 2016;71(11). https://doi.org/10.1111/all.12920.
2. P L, T.I G, H S, et al. Systemic mastocytosis patient experience from mast cell connect, the first patient-reported registry for mastocytosis. Blood 2016;128(22):4783.
3. Sokol H, Georgin-Lavialle S, Canioni D, et al. Gastrointestinal manifestations in mastocytosis: A study of 83 patients. J Allergy Clin Immunol 2013;132(4). https://doi.org/10.1016/j.jaci.2013.05.026.
4. Russell N, Jennings S, Jennings B, et al. The Mastocytosis Society Survey on Mast Cell Disorders: Part 2—Patient Clinical Experiences and Beyond. J Allergy Clin Immunol Pract 2019;7(4). https://doi.org/10.1016/j.jaip.2018.07.032.
5. Hamilton MJ, Frei SM, Stevens RL. The multifaceted mast cell in inflammatory bowel disease. Inflamm Bowel Dis 2014;20(12). https://doi.org/10.1097/MIB.0000000000000142.
6. Zhang L, Song J, Hou X. Mast cells and irritable bowel syndrome: From the bench to the bedside. J Neurogastroenterol Motil 2016;22(2). https://doi.org/10.5056/jnm15137.
7. Castells M, Austen KF. Mastocytosis: Mediator-related signs and symptoms. Int Arch Allergy Immunol 2002;127(2). https://doi.org/10.1159/000048188.
8. Cherner JA, Jensen RT, Dubois A, et al. Gastrointestinal Dysfunction in Systemic Mastocytosis: A Prospective Study. Gastroenterology 1988;95(3). https://doi.org/10.1016/S0016-5085(88)80012-X.
9. Hamilton MJ, Hornick JL, Akin C, et al. Mast cell activation syndrome: A newly recognized disorder with systemic clinical manifestations. J Allergy Clin Immunol 2011;128(1). https://doi.org/10.1016/j.jaci.2011.04.037.
10. Hamilton MJ, Zhao M, Giannetti MP, et al. Distinct Small Intestine Mast Cell Histologic Changes in Patients with Hereditary Alpha-tryptasemia and Mast Cell Activation Syndrome. Am J Surg Pathol 2021;45(7). https://doi.org/10.1097/PAS.0000000000001676.
11. Doyle LA, Sepehr GJ, Hamilton MJ, et al. A clinicopathologic study of 24 cases of systemic mastocytosis involving the gastrointestinal tract and assessment of mucosal mast cell density in irritable bowel syndrome and asymptomatic patients. Am J Surg Pathol 2014;38(6). https://doi.org/10.1097/PAS.0000000000000190.

12. Kirsch R, Geboes K, Shepherd NA, et al. Systemic mastocytosis involving the gastrointestinal tract: Clinicopathologic and molecular study of five cases. Mod Pathol 2008;21(12). https://doi.org/10.1038/modpathol.2008.158.
13. Valent P, Akin C, Escribano L, et al. Standards and standardization in mastocytosis: Consensus statements on diagnostics, treatment recommendations and response criteria. Eur J Clin Invest 2007;37(6). https://doi.org/10.1111/j.1365-2362.2007.01807.x.
14. Cardet JC, Akin C, Lee MJ. Mastocytosis: Update on pharmacotherapy and future directions. Expert Opin Pharmacother 2013;14(15). https://doi.org/10.1517/14656566.2013.824424.
15. Wasserman SI, Soter NA, Austen KF. The efficacy of oral disodium cromoglycate in human mastocytosis. J Allergy Clin Immunol 1979;63(3).
16. Gotlib J, Kluin-Nelemans HC, George TI, et al. Efficacy and Safety of Midostaurin in Advanced Systemic Mastocytosis. N Engl J Med 2016;374(26). https://doi.org/10.1056/nejmoa1513098.
17. Gotlib J, Reiter A, Radia DH, et al. Efficacy and safety of avapritinib in advanced systemic mastocytosis: interim analysis of the phase 2 PATHFINDER trial. Nat Med 2021;27(12). https://doi.org/10.1038/s41591-021-01539-8.
18. Camilleri M. Diagnosis and Treatment of Irritable Bowel Syndrome: A Review. JAMA, J Am Med Assoc 2021;325(9). https://doi.org/10.1001/jama.2020.22532.
19. Jennings S, Russell N, Jennings B, et al. The mastocytosis society survey on mast cell disorders: Patient experiences and perceptions. J Allergy Clin Immunol Pract 2014;2(1). https://doi.org/10.1016/j.jaip.2013.09.004.
20. Valent P, Akin C, Metcalfe DD, et al. 2016 updated WHO classification and novel emerging treatment concepts. Blood 2017;129(11). https://doi.org/10.1182/blood-2016-09-731893.
21. Kuruvilla ME, Mathew S, Avadhani V. Treatment of refractory mastocytic enterocolitis with budesonide. Journal of Gastrointestinal and Liver Diseases 2018;27(3). https://doi.org/10.15403/jgld.2014.1121.273.dha.
22. Mican JM, Di Bisceglie AM, Fong TL, et al. Hepatic involvement in mastocytosis: Clinicopathologic correlations in 41 cases. Hepatology 1995;22(4 PART 1). https://doi.org/10.1016/0270-9139(95)90625-8.
23. Johncilla M, Jessurun J, Brown I, et al. Are Enterocolic Mucosal Mast Cell Aggregates Clinically Relevant in Patients Without Suspected or Established Systemic Mastocytosis? Am J Surg Pathol 2018;42(10). https://doi.org/10.1097/PAS.0000000000001126.
24. Akin C, Scott LM, Kocabas CN, et al. Demonstration of an aberrant mast-cell population with clonal markers in a subset of patients with "idiopathic" anaphylaxis. Blood 2007;110(7). https://doi.org/10.1182/blood-2006-06-028100.
25. Barbara G, Stanghellini V, De Giorgio R, et al. Functional gastrointestinal disorders and mast cells: Implications for therapy. Neuro Gastroenterol Motil 2006;18(1). https://doi.org/10.1111/j.1365-2982.2005.00685.x.
26. Novak P, Giannetti MP, Weller E, et al. Mast cell disorders are associated with decreased cerebral blood flow and small fiber neuropathy. Ann Allergy Asthma Immunol 2022;128(3). https://doi.org/10.1016/j.anai.2021.10.006.
27. Wouters MM, Vicario M, Santos J. The role of mast cells in functional GI disorders. Gut 2016;65(1). https://doi.org/10.1136/gutjnl-2015-309151.
28. Hodges K, Kennedy L, Meng F, et al. Mast cells, disease and gastrointestinal cancer: A comprehensive review of recent findings. Transl Gastrointest Cancer 2012;1(2):138–50.

Management of Advanced Systemic Mastocytosis and Associated Myeloid Neoplasms

Tsewang Tashi, MD[a],*, Michael W. Deininger, MD, PhD[b]

KEYWORDS

- Systemic mastocytosis • Associated hematologic neoplasm • KIT D816 V
- KIT inhibitors • Tryptase • Avapritinib

KEY POINTS

- Advanced systemic mastocytosis (AdvSM) is a heterogeneous group of disorders characterized by neoplastic mast cell-related organ damage and frequently associated with a myeloid neoplasm.
- KIT D816V, a gain-of-function mutation and the primary oncogenic driver, is found in about 90% of all patients with AdvSM.
- Midostaurin—an oral multikinase inhibitor, and avapritinib—a selective KIT inhibitor, are approved therapies for AdvSM.
- Avapritinib provides deeper and more durable responses compared to midostaurin in treating the mastocytosis component, but its effect on the associated hematologic neoplasm (AHN) is unclear.
- Future studies are needed to evaluate combination therapies of KIT inhibitors with different AHN treatments.

INTRODUCTION

Systemic mastocytosis (SM) is a rare hematologic malignancy characterized by aberrant proliferation and accumulation of clonal mast cells (MC) in one or more extracutaneous organs or tissues. Mutational activation of KIT is central to SM pathogenesis, with *KIT* D816V accounting for more than 90% of KIT mutations found in SM.[1,2] Depending on the extent of the organ involvement and its effects on organ function, SM is classified into indolent systemic mastocytosis (ISM), smoldering systemic mastocytosis (SSM) and advanced systemic mastocytosis (AdvSM). AdvSM encompasses

[a] Division of Hematology and Hematologic Malignancies, Huntsman Cancer Institute, University of Utah, 2000, Circle of Hope, Salt Lake City, UT 84112, USA; [b] Division of Hematology and Oncology, Medical College of Wisconsin, Versiti Blood Research Institute, 8727 West Watertown Plank Road, Milwaukee, WI 53226, USA
* Corresponding author.
E-mail address: tsewang.tashi@utah.edu

Immunol Allergy Clin N Am 43 (2023) 723–741
https://doi.org/10.1016/j.iac.2023.04.009
0889-8561/23/© 2023 Elsevier Inc. All rights reserved.

immunology.theclinics.com

aggressive SM (ASM), SM with associated hematologic neoplasm (SM-AHN) and mast cell leukemia (MCL). End-organ damage and/or compromised function as a result of MC infiltration are referred to as "C-findings."

Prior to the approval in 2017 of midostaurin, a multikinase inhibitor with activity against KIT D816V, cladribine and interferon-α (IFNα) were commonly used in the treatment of AdvSM. However, these treatments were associated with limited efficacy and high toxicity.[3,4] In a phase 2 study of patients with AdvSM, midostaurin had an overall response (OR) rate of 60%.[5,6] Although most responses were partial and not durable, and there was significant gastrointestinal toxicity, this was a significant improvement in the treatment of AdvSM.[7] Recently, avapritinib, a selective and potent inhibitor of KIT D816 V, was approved for the treatment of AdvSM. Avapritnib was highly effective in reducing bone marrow (BM) MC burden, KIT D816V allele frequency, and serum tryptase level.[8–12] In phase 1 and 2 studies, OR rates were 75% to 85% with complete response (CR) rates of 32% to 36%. Adverse events were much more manageable compared with midostaurin. Bezuclastinib and elenestinib are 2 additional novel KIT D816V tyrosine kinase inhibitors (TKI) currently in clinical trials.[13,14] Preliminary results show promising efficacy in treating SM, but more follow-up is needed to determine how these TKIs compare to avapritinib. In this review, we will first introduce the pathophysiology, clinical features and diagnosis of AdvSM, then discuss the management of AdvSM and the associated hematological malignancies.

PATHOPHYSIOLOGY, CLINICAL FEATURES, AND DIAGNOSIS OF ADVANCED SYSTEMIC MASTOCYTOSIS
KIT Mutations in Advanced Systemic Mastocytosis

KIT is the transmembrane receptor for stem cell factor (SCF) and belongs to the class III family of receptor tyrosine kinases. It plays a central role in the growth, differentiation, maturation, and survival of normal MC.[15,16] Spanning 976 amino acids, KIT is organized into extracellular, transmembrane, and intracellular domains. The intracellular domain comprises a juxtamembrane and a split kinase domain separated by a kinase insert.[15] A gain-of-function mutation in the kinase domain, D816 V, is found in more than 90% of SM cases.[2] Several much less common but functionally equivalent point mutations in codon 816 have been described.[1] KIT D816V confers ligand-independent activation of KIT and its downstream signaling pathways, including phosphatidylinositol 3-kinase (PI3K), mitogen-activated protein kinase (MAPK), and Janus kinase/signal transducer and activator of transcription (STAT) pathways. In aggregate, these pathways promote MC proliferation, differentiation, and survival.[15]

In a subset of cases of AdvSM, the KIT D816V mutation is restricted to MCs, whereas in others its presence is demonstrable in other myeloid cells, consistent with multilineage involvement.[17,18] Single-cell studies from patients with SM have suggested that the acquisition of KIT D816V is an early event in the hematopoietic stem and progenitor cell (HSPC) compartment,[19] which drives HSPC to favor MC differentiation. In contrast, in non-MC myeloid lineage cells, the acquisition of KIT D816V may be a secondary event.[20] Multilineage involvement by KIT D816V is more evident in AdvSM with higher KIT variant allele frequency (VAF) at presentation.[20–22]

Interestingly, KIT mutations, including D816V, have been described frequently in core binding factor acute myeloid luekemia (CBF-AML)—those that harbor t(8;21) or inv(16) or t(16;16). In these cases, the bone marrow (BM) does not always show morphologic evidence of mastocytosis.[23,24] It is unknown whether this represents a unique entity or there are mast cell aggregates that escaped detection due to sampling errors or whether the two diseases co-exist.[25–27] CBF-AML is generally categorized into favorable risk group but the presence of *KIT* D816 is associated with adverse prognosis.[28,29] However, now that the *KIT* D816V can be targeted with inhibitors, prognostic relevance may no longer be the same, and perhaps even favorable. Indeed, a recent small case series from China demonstrated a rapid and deep response to avapritinib in *KIT*-mutated CBF-AML.[24]

Various mutationss have been identified in the extracellular, transmembrane, and juxtamembrane domains of the *KIT* gene, but these are much less common and usually associated with sensitivity to imatinib. *KIT* mutations other than D816V are typical of gastrointestinal stromal tumors (GIST), and are sometimes seen in melanoma.[30–34]

Clinical Features and Diagnosis of Advanced Systemic Mastocytosis

Patients with SM often present with symptoms related to mediator release through MC degranulation. These symptoms include rash, flushing, diarrhea, nausea, vomiting, dizziness, headaches, and brain fog, among others. Life-threatening anaphylaxis can occasionally occur in response to specific triggers such as certain foods, medications, and even physical or emotional stress.[35] These are more common in patients with ISM where symptom improvement remains the primary goal of therapy. In AdvSM, mediator-release symptoms may still occur; however, patients often present with consequences of organ damage from infiltration of neoplastic MC (C-findings, **Box 1**),[36] and/or an AHN that may cause abnormal blood counts.

The diagnosis of SM is based on WHO diagnostic criteria, which include 1 major and 4 minor criteria and were last updated in 2022.[37] These updated diagnostic criteria for SM are the same in the recent International Consensus Classification (ICC), which was developed separately and independently of WHO by the Society of Hematopathology and the European Association of Haematopathology, based on inputs from clinical advisory committees from around the world.[38] The major criterion is the presence of multifocal dense aggregates of MC (>15 cells per aggregate) in the BM or on any extracutaneous biopsy. Minor criteria include spindle-shaped morphology of at least 25% of the MC, aberrant expression of CD2, CD25, and/or CD30 by the neoplastic MC, presence of any activating *KIT* mutation, and increased serum tryptase level (>20 μg/L; **Box 2**). One major and 1 minor criterion, or 3 minor criteria, are required to establish a diagnosis of SM.[38,39] Although any extracutaneous biopsy showing aggregates of aberrant MC fulfills the major criterion, BM is almost always involved in AdvSM. Consequently, a BM biopsy is required to evaluate both for neoplastic MC

Box 1
C-findings for advanced systemic mastocytosis

There have been no changes to the C-findings in both the updated 5th edition (2022) WHO diagnostic criteria and ICC criteria for SM. At least one C-finding is required for the diagnosis of AdvSM.
1. Bone marrow dysfunction caused by MC infiltration, causing cytopenia(s): Absolute neutrophil count less than 1×10^9/L, Hb < 10 g/dL or platelets less than 100×10^9/L)
2. Hepatomegaly with impairment of liver function, ascites, and/or portal hypertension
3. Palpable splenomegaly with hypersplenism (platelet < 100×10^9/L)
4. Gastrointestinal MC infiltrates causing malabsorption with weight loss greater than 10%
5. Skeletal involvement with large osteosclerotic or lytic lesion (>2 cm) or with pathologic fractures due to the lesions.

Data from DeAngelo DJ, Radia DH, George TI, et al. Safety and efficacy of avapritinib in advanced systemic mastocytosis: the phase 1 EXPLORER trial. Nat Med. 2021;27(12):2183-2191.

Box 2
Diagnostic criteria for systemic mastocytosis

(One major and 1 minor criterion; or 3 minor criteria are required for establishing a diagnosis of SM)

The 5th edition (2022) WHO diagnostic criteria and ICC criteria for systemic mastocytosis

Major Criterion:
1. Multifocal, dense aggregates of MC (>15 cells) in the bone marrow or other extracutaneous biopsy

Minor Criteria:
1. More than 25% of the MC have aberrant spindled-shaped morphology
2. Mast cell express CD117 and CD2, CD25 and/or CD30
3. Positive for any activating *KIT* mutation
4. Serum tryptase greater than 20 μg/L (not applicable for SM-AHN)

1. The inclusion of CD30 as a marker of aberrant MC and any activating *KIT* mutations are the notable changes in the 2022 WHO criteria compared to the 2016 WHO criteria.

Data from Khoury JD, Solary E, Abla O, et al. The 5th edition of the World Health Organization Classification of Haematolymphoid Tumours: Myeloid and Histiocytic/Dendritic Neoplasms. Leukemia. 2022;36(7):1703-1719.

---

and for the potential presence of an AHN. Detection of a *KIT* mutation is a crucial part of the diagnostic work-up, although a small portion of SM are *KIT* wild type. Many reference laboratories have developed highly sensitive digital PCR tests for the KIT *D816V* mutation that can detect variant alleles down to 0.02% VAF.[40] Additionally, we recommend next-generation sequencing of genes associated with myeloid malignancies in all patients with AdvSM. This is not only useful for the initial evaluation of potential AHN, but also for prognostication and monitoring of clonal evolution during treatment.

Serum tryptase should be measured in all patients suspected of SM. Tryptase is almost always elevated in SM such that tryptase greater than 20 μg/L is one of the minor criteria per WHO diagnostic criteria.[37,39] Although the levels vary greatly among different types of SM and even between individuals,[41] it often exceeds 200 μg/L in AdvSM, and is one of the independent prognostic markers in the International Prognostic Scoring System for Mastocytosis (IPSM).[42]

Elevated tryptase levels can be seen in several conditions, particularly in myeloid neoplasms such as AML, MDS, and chronic myeloid leukemia (CML).[43] Another important differential diagnosis to consider for patients with elevated serum tryptase is hereditary alpha tryptasemia (HaT)—a rare genetic condition where an extra copy of the alpha-tryptase gene is inherited.[44] Clinical significance of HaT is still being investigated, but it is thought to represent a factor in augmenting the severity of allergic reactions in patients with venom allergies and possibly in patients with mastocytosis. HaT can occur concurrently with SM, and in fact, the prevalence of HaT was reported to be higher among patients with SM.[45] In current clinical practice, we do not test for HaT upfront but do recommend testing for it in 2 scenarios: (1) if the initial work-up does not reveal SM, and (2) if serum tryptase level does not normalize despite effective KIT inhibitor therapy in patients with SM.

An elevated level of MC mediators, such as serum histamine levels, and its urine metabolite, N-methylhistamine is well established in SM but lacks specificity as it can be elevated in nonclonal mast cell activation syndrome (MCAS) and carcinoids.[46] Moreover, the levels varied considerably among individuals and with the timing of sample collection with respect to mediator symptom episodes, making these tests quite unreliable and of little practical utility. Given the relative ease of obtaining morphologic evidence of aberrant MC, and with the incorporation of *KIT* mutation and serum tryptase in the WHO diagnostic criteria, testing serum histamine or its urine metabolites is not part of our routine SM diagnostic work-up. However, they may have a role in those patients who do not have SM, but still have MC mediator-release symptoms and are suspected to have idiopathic MCAS.

After establishing the diagnosis of SM, the burden of clonal MC and potential C-findings must be assessed. We suggest the following diagnostic approach.

- Complete blood count (CBC) with differential: CBC may show elevated or reduced blood counts, which may reflect either MC infiltration, AHN, or both. Cytopenias can also result from hypersplenism, or from prior cytotoxic therapies.
- Chemistry panel including liver function tests (LFT): AnElevated LFTs, especially elevated alkaline phosphatase, suggests MC infiltration of the liver. If the patient has preexisting liver disease, and MC involvement is highly suspected, a liver biopsy may be needed for confirmation. Low serum albumin may reflect malnutrition resulting from gastrointestinal MC involvement.
- Abdominal ultrasound or CT/MRI to evaluate for hepatomegaly, splenomegaly, and lymphadenopathy.
- Bone density scan and skeletal survey to evaluate for osteoporosis and bone lesions. The high prevalence of osteopenia/osteoporosis and sclerotic/lytic bone lesions in patients with SM is thought to reflect the effects of MC mediators and cytokines on the bone remodeling process.[47]

The presence of any one C-finding suffices for establishing a diagnosis of AdvSM. An exception is MCL, where C-findings are frequently found, though not required for diagnosis.[36,37]

Classification of Advanced Systemic Mastocytosis

SM-AHN comprises about 70% to 75% of all AdvSM.[9] Most of the AHN cases are myeloid in origin. Chronic myelomonocytic leukemia (CMML) is the most common, representing about 40% of AHNs. Others include myelodysplastic syndrome (MDS), myeloproliferative neoplasms (MPN), chronic eosinophilic leukemia (CEL), MDS/MPN-unclassifiable, and AML. Lymphoid neoplasms, such as chronic lymphocytic leukemia, Hodgkin's and non-Hodgkin's lymphoma, and multiple myeloma, is occasionally seen in association with SM, but is thought to have a different clonal origin. The presence of premalignant conditions, such as monoclonal gammopathy or monoclonal B-cell lymphocytosis, does not qualify as AHN. Unlike the 2022 WHO classification, which continues to use the term "SM-AHN," the recent ICC criteria for myeloid neoplasms has renamed SM-AHN as "SM-associated myeloid neoplasm" (AMN),[39] effectively excluding lymphoid neoplasms as AHN.

AHN can present as subtle abnormalities on BM morphology. Molecular and cytogenetic data are often helpful for evaluating the potential AHN. For example, mutations in *SRSF2*, *ASXL1*, *TET2*, and/or the RAS pathway may point to an underlying CMML or MDS/MPN, whereas mutations in *JAK2*, *CALR*, or *CSF3R* point to an underlying MPN. In patients with eosinophilia, it is important to screen for *PDGRFα/β*, *FGFR1*, and *JAK2* rearrangements, as these belong to a separate entity in the WHO myeloid disease classification—myeloid/lymphoid neoplasms with eosinophilia and rearrangement of *PDGFRA*, *PDGFRB*, or *FGFR1*, or with *PCM1-JAK2*. Eosinophilia can also be seen in other chronic myeloid neoplasms; therefore, a detailed review of the BM, along with cytogenetics and molecular data by an experienced hematopathologist, is important in identifying the correct diagnosis. It is worthwhile to note that in avapritinib studies, KIT inhibition resulted in prompt normalization of peripheral and BM eosino-philia in patients with SM-CEL,[10,48] suggesting perhaps a common KIT driver. In fact, *KIT* D816V has been demonstrated in eosinophils indicating that eosinophils are part of the multilineage clone.[49] Missense mutations in *ETNK1* are enriched in SM present-ing with eosinophilia, and also in CMML and atypical CML,[50,51] but their functional consequences are largely unknown.

ASM, which comprises about 25% of AdvSM, predominantly manifests with symp-toms from C-findings, that is, MC-associated organ infiltration and damage, such as hepatosplenomegaly, pleural effusions and/or ascites, lymphadenopathy, GI involve-ment causing diarrhea leading to malabsorption, skeletal involvement with pathologic fractures related to osteosclerosis, osteolysis, or osteoporosis. A biopsy of involved organs will show aberrant spindled-shaped MC. If the neoplastic MC in the BM smear is greater than 5%, the term "ASM in transformation" to MCL (ASM-t) can be used to indicate a high risk of progression to secondary MCL.[37]

MCL is very rare, accounting for less than 5% of all mastocytosis cases, and has the worst prognosis among all AdvSM subtypes with a median overall survival (OS) of less than 2 years.[52] Patients often present with constitutional symptoms of night sweats, weight loss, and fatigue in addition to the C-findings that may or may not be present.[37] In addition to fulfilling the WHO diagnostic criteria for SM, the diagnosis requires greater than 20% spindled-shaped clonal MC in the BM aspirate. MCL can be classi-fied into different variants depending on presentation and clinical course. Acute MCL typically has an aggressive course, and C-findings are often seen at presentation, whereas chronic MCL has a more indolent course and lacks C-findings. Although chronic MCL has a better prognosis compared to acute MCL, many of these patients progress over time. MCL can also be divided into classical (leukemic variant, >10% MC in the peripheral blood) and aleukemic variant (<10% MC in the peripheral blood). MCL can be either *de novo* or secondary to preexisting ASM and may or may not have an AHN component. The primary differential diagnosis includes myelomastocytic leu-kemia (MML), a rare myeloid neoplasm with partial MC differentiation.[36] Unlike the neoplastic MC in MCL, the leukemic blasts in MML are typically immature and myelo-blastic, expressing CD34 and weak CD117, and are negative for *KIT* mutations.

MANAGEMENT OF ADVANCED SYSTEMIC MASTOCYTOSIS

Unlike ISM, where the goal of therapy is symptom improvement, the management of AdvSM can be broadly categorized into 3 aspects: reducing clonal MC, alleviating mediator symptoms, and managing the AHN component if present. As AdvSM is char-acterized by MC-associated organ damage (C-finding), treating to prevent further damage, and attempting to reverse the damage through cytoreduction are the objec-tives of therapy. Before the advent of targeted therapies, recombinant interferon-α (IFNα) and cytotoxic chemotherapies such as cladribine were commonly used but had limited efficacy.[3,4,53] With the approval of midostaurin in 2017,[6] and the recent development of selective KIT inhibitors such as avapritinib,[9] there is a significant advancement in the treatment of AdvSM with much-improved efficacy and outcome. At the same time, these new and effective treatments have also provided us with deeper insights into the natural history of clonal evolution, especially in patients with SM-AHN. We will review these treatment approaches in the following sections.

Treatment of Mediator Release Symptoms

Mediator symptoms from MC degranulation are more common in patients with ISM and SSM but can also occur in patients with AdvSM. Such symptoms can be debilitating and significantly affect the quality of life, sometimes more than organ damage does. Treatment strategies for mediator symptoms are similar to ISM management, including H1/H2 receptor blockers, leukotriene inhibitors, MC stabilizers (eg, cromolyn sodium and ketotifen), IgE monoclonal antibodies (eg, omalizumab), and corticosteroids.[54] Although most patients require multiple agents to control symptoms, therapy is highly individualized since mediator symptoms vary greatly between patients.

Nonsedating second-generation H1 receptor blockers, such as loratadine, cetirizine, and fexofenadine, are usually the first line of therapy, and patients often require higher than conventional over-the-counter doses. First-generation H1 receptor blockers such as diphenhydramine and hydroxyzine are typically reserved for breakthrough symptoms or emergent situations because of their sedating effect and shorter half-life. H2 receptor blockers such as famotidine and MC stabilizers are more helpful for patients with gastrointestinal symptoms. We recommend maximizing the dose of one agent in a stepwise approach before considering additional agents. Besides medications, avoiding known triggers is essential to preventing mediator-release symptoms. Anti-IgE therapy may benefit patients with concurrent asthma.

Reduction of Mast Cell Burden

Interferon-α and cladribine
Before the approval of midostaurin, no standard therapy existed for AdvSM, and the 2 most commonly used agents were IFNα and cladribine.[4,53,55] Although IFNα is effective in certain myeloproliferative neoplasms, such as CML, polycythemia vera, and essential thrombocythemia, its efficacy in SM is quite limited. The only prospective study was a phase II trial of 20 patients (17 AdvSM, 3 ISM) that showed a 35% partial response rate and no complete response in patients receiving IFNα.[53] In particular, no responses were noted in patients who had organomegaly or cytopenia at enrollment, and the incidence of treatment-associated depression was high at 35%. IFNα is generally poorly tolerated compared to the newer, longer-acting pegylated IFNα, but there are no studies of pegylated IFNα in SM.

Cladribine is a nucleoside analog and is often a part of acute leukemia treatment regimens. Based on historical case series, response rates with cladribine in AdvSM have been around 50% to 77%, with no complete responses and median response duration ranging from 10 to 30 months.[3,55,56] However, cladribine is associated with significant cytopenias and prolonged suppression of T-cell immunity, rendering patients vulnerable to life-threatening fungal and opportunistic infections. In several case series, one-third to half of the patients had grade 3/4 neutropenia, and more than three-fourths had prolonged lymphopenia.[3,55,56]

With the approval of midostaurin and, more recently avapritinib, cladribine, and IFNα are of mostly historical interest. Cladribine may still have an indication, for instance, as salvage therapy in rare refractory cases of AdvSM requiring immediate cytoreduction. Although combining with a KIT inhibitor is an attractive option, combination therapy has not been studied.

KIT-targeted tyrosine kinase inhibitors
Imatinib. Imatinib was developed to treat CML by inhibiting ABL kinase activity by competing with ATP binding to the catalytic site, ushering in the era of molecular targeted therapy in cancer treatment.[57] In addition to the ABL kinase inhibition, imatinib showed inhibitory activity against PDGFR and KIT tyrosine kinases,[58] leading to its use in SM. Early small prospective studies and case series failed to show clinically significant efficacy in patients with KIT D816V-positive SM but showed some activity in KIT D816V-negative patients.[59–61] These clinical observations led to the FDA approval of

imatinib in 2006 for SM in patients negative for *KIT* D816V or with unknown *KIT* mutation status. Subsequent *in vitro* studies showed that imatinib inhibits the growth of MC with wild-type *KIT* or with mutations outside the exon 17 activation loop,[62] whereas the D816V mutation confers resistance because of a conformational change in the catalytic pocket.[63] In current clinical practice, we reserve imatinib for patients with wild-type *KIT* or those that harbor mutations outside of the kinase domain.[64]

Midostaurin. Midostaurin is an ATP-competitive broad-spectrum TKI with activity against the receptor kinases of fms-related receptor tyrosine kinase 3 (FLT3), fibroblast growth factor receptor (FGFR), protein kinase C, and KIT among others.[65] It gained FDA approval in 2017 for AdvSM based on a phase 2 open-label study of 116 patients, which showed an overall response rate (ORR) of 59.6% based on the 89 patients with at least one evaluable C-finding.[6] Among the responders, about 45% of the patients had a major response (defined as resolution of one or more C-findings), and 15% achieved a partial response. Dividing by the subtypes, the ORR was 75% for ASM, 57.9% for SM-AHN, and 50% for MCL. Toxicity requiring dose reduction occurred in 56% of the patients. The most frequent adverse events were GI symptoms, including nausea, vomiting, and diarrhea. Myelosuppression was common, with grade 3/4 (G3/4) neutropenia in 24%, G3/4 anemia in 41%, and G3/4 thrombocytopenia in 29%. In a more recent post hoc analysis, 113 of 116 patients had a C-finding per modified International Working Group-Myeloproliferative Neoplasm Research and Treatment & European Competence Network on Mastocytosis (mIWG-MRT-ECNM) response criteria, and the ORR was 28.3%. In this analysis, ORR was 60% for ASM, 20.8% for SM-AHN, and 33.3% for MCL.[6] A phase 2 study of midostaurin in 26 patients with AdvSM followed for a median of 10 years showed a median OS of 40 months, with 2 patients achieving complete response (CR) at 12 months and beyond.[5] The approved midostaurin dose in AdvSM is 100 mg twice daily, in contrast to 50 mg twice daily for AML with a FLT3 mutation. Gastrointestinal and hematological toxicities, together with overall limited clinical activity (median OS in the phase 2 study was 28.7 months), have limited the use of midostaurin as the first-line treatment in AdvSM, particularly since the approval of avapritinib. With more potent and specific KIT inhibitors in the pipeline, the use of midostaurin is likely to decline even further.

Avapritinib. Avapritinib is a potent KIT inhibitor with selective activity against the KIT and the structurally similar PDGFRα/β kinase.[66] It was evaluated in 2 open-label single-arm studies: the phase 1 EXPLORER study and the phase 2 PATHFINDER study. The EXPLORER study included 69 patients with AdvSM treated at doses of 30 to 400 mg. In the 53 response evaluable patients, ORR was 75% with a CR rate of 36%, and 92% of the patients achieved greater than 50% reduction in BM MC. In more than 80% of the patients, *KIT* D816V VAF decreased by more than 50% from baseline and became undetectable in 30%, measured by digital droplet polymerase chain reaction (ddPCR) with a limit of detection of 0.17%. Reduction in *KIT* D816V VAF also correlated with the depth of clinical response. The most common adverse events were periorbital edema, nausea, diarrhea, anemia, and thrombocytopenia. Intracranial hemorrhage occurred in 9 (13%) patients, with a platelet count of less than 50×10^9/L in all but one patient.[48] Although cognitive and memory impairment can be features of SM, these were not as common as reported in avapritinib studies in GIST patients.[67] The recommended phase 2 dosing for the ongoing PATHFINDER study was 200 mg. Preliminary results from PATHFINDER, which included 107 patients with AdvSM, continue to show good efficacy with ORR of 84%, with 32%

CR/CRh and 48% achieving a partial response (PR) across all AdvSM subtypes and OS of 88% at 2 years, using the mIWG-MRT-ECNM response criteria. Most common adverse events were similar to the EXPLORER study, except that no intracranial bleeding has been reported thus far.[10] In a recent pooled analysis of avapritinib in the EXPLORER and PATHFINDER studies in patients who had received one prior systemic treatment (n = 31), the ORR was 71%, with a 19% CR/CRh rate.[12]

Based on these findings from phase 1 and 2 studies, avapritinib was approved for AdvSM in the United States by the FDA in 2021 and in Europe by EMA in 2022 for patients with at least 1 prior therapy. It is the first selective KIT inhibitor to be approved for AdvSM. With its improved efficacy and tolerance, it is likely to replace midostaurin as the first line of therapy.

Ongoing KIT inhibitor trials. Bezuclastinib is a novel potent KIT inhibitor currently being evaluated in AdvSM in the ongoing APEX trial. Early results have been very encouraging, including reduction of BM MC, serum tryptase levels, and *KIT* D816V VAF.[14] Elenestinib (BLU-263) is another potent KIT inhibitor and is being evaluated in AdvSM, both as monotherapy and in combination with HMA in patients with AHN progression.[68]

Unlike avapritinib, preclinical studies in these novel selective KIT inhibitors claim minimal activity against related kinases such as PDGFR, FGFR, and FLT3, thereby mitigating off-target effects. They also suggest minimal penetration across the blood-brain barrier, potentially mitigating central nervous system effects.[13,69] This may alleviate concerns about cognitive impairment in all and intracranial hemorrhage in patients with low platelet counts taking avapritinib.

Immunotherapy directed against cell surface antigens. Neoplastic MC express several cell surface antigens, including CD2, CD25, and CD30. Although no available drugs target CD2 or CD25, CD30 can be targeted using brentuximab vedotin. However, a phase II trial of brentuximab vedotin monotherapy in AdvSM failed to show any meaningful response.[70]

Management of Associated Hematologic Neoplasms

Although the emergence of potent KIT inhibitors has changed the therapeutic landscape of SM by inducing deeper and more durable responses than prior therapies, its effect on the AHN component remains uncertain. Response assessments in the KIT inhibitor trials in AdvSM have been mainly focused on the SM endpoints using the mIWG-MRT-ECNM response criteria.[6,10,14] As the AHN component is assessed per AHN-specific response for the relevant myeloid neoplasm if the AHN progresses requiring therapy, patients have to come off the study, even if the SM component continues to respond. This and the difficulty distinguishing between drug-induced myelosuppression and disease-related cytopenia make the interpretation of results challenging and impact overall efficacy analysis.

In the midostaurin trial in patients with AdvSM, with a median follow-up of 26 months, the rate of leukemic transformation was 11% (n = 13).[6] Jawhar and colleagues[71] reported in their analysis of a subset of 38 patients (20 on midostaurin trial and 18 on expanded access use) disease progression to MCL or leukemic transformation in 6 out of 38 patients (16%); and in 5/6 (83%) patients, the disease evolved from preexisting SM-AHN within a median time of 14 months. These progressions were associated with (i) the presence of at least one mutation in *SRSF2, ASXL1,* or *RUNX1 (S/A/R)*, (ii) increasing VAF of preexisting mutations, or (iii) development of new mutations in *K/NRAS, RUNX1,* and *IDH2* genes despite a reduction in *KIT*

D816V VAF. In the EXPLORER study of avapritinib, in 69 evaluable patients, with a median follow-up of 23 months, the rate of clinical progression was 20% (n = 14), of which 10/48 (21%) were patients with SM-AHN whose AHN progressed and 4/13 (31%) with MCL progression. These progressions were associated with the acquisition of mutations in *NRAS, GATA2, SRSF2, NPM1, SETBP1,* or *CBL*, indicating clonal evolution. Similar to the midostaurin-treated SM-AHN cases, the AHN progression was not associated with increased *KIT* D816V VAF.[72] A recent single-cell DNA study on a patient with SM-CMML treated with midostaurin also showed that AHN clonal progression occurred independent of *KIT* D816V mutation.[73]

Although complete data for the rate of AHN progression in the ongoing KIT inhibitor trials are still forthcoming, some general observations can be made: First, despite the excellent molecular response of the SM component, KIT inhibition does not seem to have the same impact of response on the AHN component, suggesting that even in case of multilineage involvement by *KIT* D816V, this mutation is often not the main driver of the AHN component. However, the initial KIT inhibition in the AHN component may still delay progression, as suggested by the reduction of monocytosis in SM-CMML early in the treatment with avapritinib.[10,48] Second, certain preexisting somatic mutations, such as *S/A/R* mutations, are associated with a high risk of progression. Third, under the selective pressure of KIT inhibition, clonal progression of the AHN is often KIT-independent (**Fig. 1**).

Treatment approaches for AHN and its responses are highly variable depending on the type of AHN. Whether to treat the SM first or the AHN first depends on the primary cause of the clinical symptoms and the organ damage (C-findings). In clinical practice, it is often difficult to determine whether symptoms are from the SM or the AHN component. However, given that SM treatment with a selective KIT inhibitor is much more convenient and effective than treatment of MDS, MDS/MPN, or CMML with hypomethylating agents, it seems quite reasonable to start SM treatment and assess symptom improvement for causal attribution. In these patients, close monitoring of the *KIT* D816V VAF and extended mutation panel by next-generation sequencing (NGS) should be done to track the AHN more closely. If the AHN is a high-grade myeloid neoplasm, such as AML, MDS with excess blasts, or a high-risk MPN, then AHN treatment will typically take precedence or one may need to treat both SM and AHN components concurrently.

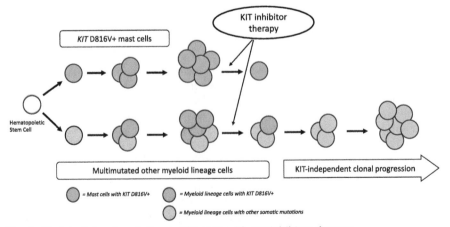

Fig. 1. Model of clonal evolution in SM-AHN with KIT inhibitor therapy.

Challenges in the Management of Associated Hematologic Neoplasms

There is a dearth of data for combining KIT inhibitors with other antineoplastic agents in patients with SM-AHN. Increased myelosuppression remains one of the primary concerns. As such, future studies are needed to assess the safety and optimal dosing of such combination therapies. An adaptive basket trial design with a KIT inhibitor backbone combined with different treatments for different AHN arms could be an option,[74] but with SM and AHN progressing at their own respective pace, conducting such a trial would be quite challenging. In the absence of safety data, when combining available therapies with KIT inhibitors, it would be prudent to start both agents at a lower dose to assess tolerability and then gradually titrate to the optimal dose with close monitoring. These patients should be referred to and treated at an academic medical center with expertise in SM management.

In current clinical practice, AHN is treated when it shows signs of clinical progression (eg, the development of significant cytopenia and an increase in BM blast count). Although this treatment strategy is consistent with current standard approaches for CMML, MDS, or MDS/MPN without SM, the question remains whether this is the best approach in SM-AHN. One thought would be that AHN treatment may be initiated when the SM component achieves a complete pathologic response (eg, when *KIT* D816V becomes undetectable or abnormal BM MCs are no longer seen) instead of waiting until AHN shows signs of clinical progression. Further studies are needed to determine whether results would be improved based on the timing of initiating treatment.

Allogeneic stem cell transplantation (alloSCT) remains an important treatment option for patients with AdvSM, especially in patients with SM-AHN and MCL at progression. However, there has not been any prospective study so far, and the largest retrospective study published in 2014 consisted of only 57 patients (SM-AHN = 38; ASM = 7; MCL = 12). ORR for the SM component was 70%, with 28% achieving CR. For the AHN component, there was 100% CR in all 38 patients with SM-AHN, but the AHN subsequently relapsed in 26% of patients. Three-year OS was 57% for all patients (74% for SM-AHN, 43% for ASM, and 17% for MCL). Adverse prognostic factors were MCL diagnosis and the use of a reduced-intensity conditioning regimen.[75]

Currently, there are no guidelines for the optimal timing or the conditioning approach for alloSCT in AdvSM. However, early consideration for transplant should be given in AdvSM, particularly in (i) acute MCL, (ii) SM-AHN, when AHN shows signs of clonal evolution with the emergence of high-risk cytogenetics and molecular features, and if the AHN is a high-risk myeloid neoplasm, such as AML, high-grade MDS, or MDS/MPN with excess blasts.[76] With the encouraging results of KIT inhibition inducing durable CR in the SM component, indication and timing for alloSCT are increasingly driven primarily by clonal evolution and progression of the AHN component. In certain ASM and chronic MCL without AHN, where KIT is the sole primary driver of the disease, perhaps one could argue that alloSCT should be delayed, possibly even until signs of progression are detected.

PROGNOSTIC MARKERS IN ADVANCED SYSTEMIC MASTOCYTOSIS

AdvSM generally has a much shorter survival compared with ISM, but the prognosis varies greatly between the 3 subtypes of AdvSM. In a single institution retrospective study of 183 patients with AdvSM with 21 months median follow-up, ASM had the longest median OS with 41 months, followed by SM-AHN with 24 months, and MCL had the shortest median OS with 2 months.[77] In patients with SM-AHN, median OS also varied with the type of AHN, with the longest median OS of 31 months in patients who had an MPN and the shortest median OS of 11 months with AML.[78] Considering the molecular abnormalities, S/A/R mutations are associated with inferior survival (ORR 39%, vs. 75% in those without S/A/R mutation), and response to midostaurin with greater than 25% reduction in KIT D816 V allele burden was associated with superior OS.[71,79,80]

Over the last several years, several prognostic scoring systems have been developed in SM, each comprising clinical, laboratory, and molecular parameters found to have prognostic significance. In both Mayo Alliance Prognostic System (MAPS) and Mutation-Adjusted Risk Score (MARS) for AdvSM, age greater than 60 years, the presence of high molecular risk gene mutations (NRAS, ASXL1, and/or RUNX1 in MAPS; S/A/R in MARS), anemia with hemoglobin of less than 10 g/dL, and thrombocytopenia with platelet count less than 100×10^9/L were shown to be independent risk factors for OS on multivariate analysis.[81,82] The International Prognostic Scoring System for Mastocytosis (IPSM), based on the largest cohort of 1639 patients with SM in the ECNM registry, additionally identified tryptase greater than 125 µg/L, WBC greater than 16×10^9/L, and lack of skin involvement as adverse prognostic factors in AdvSM.[42] However, most of these were cladribine and midostaurin-treated patients. With the arrival of avapritinib and other selective KIT inhibitors in the pipeline, providing higher hematologic response rates, durable KIT inhibition, and robust decline of tryptase levels, these risk models and prognostic markers need to be reevaluated and validated in future cohorts treated with KIT inhibitors.

Response Assessments of Systemic Mastocytosis and Associated Hematologic Neoplasm and their Challenges

MC-related organ damage is the defining feature of AdvSM. Response assessment criteria were developed successively by different groups, including Valent and colleagues in 2003, the Mayo Clinic in 2010, and the combined IWG-MRT-ECNM networks in 2013. All are anchored mainly in the reversal of one or more C-finding.[82–84] The IWG-MRT-ECNM criteria are the most comprehensive, including clinical, histopathological, and laboratory parameters, providing more granularity to the definitions of MC-related organ damage and their clinical responses. However, since the system was established with the intent to harmonize adjudication of responses for patients in clinical trials, the response criteria required quantifiable MC-related organ damage to facilitate objective assessment of changes on treatment. This has led to differences between the WHO-defined C-findings, and the MC-related organ damages that are eligible for response assessment. For example, large osteosclerotic/lytic lesions and associated pathologic fractures are excluded from the IWG response criteria since quantifying these is quite challenging. Although splenomegaly with hypersplenism is a WHO-defined C-finding, the presence of only splenomegaly (>5 cm below left costal margin) qualifies as eligible organ damage for IWG response assessment. Furthermore, vulnerabilities were exposed in the interpretation and quantification of some of the WHO-defined C-findings, such as malabsorption and weight loss, as weight changes are often not well documented and can also be confounded by fluid shifts.[85,86]

In practice, the application of IWG response criteria can be challenging, especially in SM-AHN, where either the SM or AHN component can lead to organ damage and/or cytopenia. In some cases, organ damage and/or cytopenia can be confounded by the effects of ongoing therapy, toxicity, or other comorbidities, and a biopsy of the affected organ can be needed for confirmation of a causal relationship to SM. This is reflected in the modified IWG-MRT-ECNM criteria, where a category of CRh (CR with partial hematologic recovery) is included to account for lingering cytopenia that may be from factors other than SM. Furthermore, as SM-AHN and MCL do not always require WHO-defined C-findings for diagnosis, applying response criteria in these circumstances becomes impossible. In the KIT inhibitor clinical trials, these patients have often been stratified in a separate cohort as having "unevaluable IWG response criteria."

Given these challenges and complexities of IWG-MRT-ECNM criteria, pure pathologic response (PPR) criteria, based on the objective histopathologic response achieved, have been proposed. They include assessments of BM MC burden along with laboratory parameters, including changes in serum tryptase level and complete or partial hematologic response. Elimination of BM MC aggregates, serum tryptase less than 20 µg/L, and a complete or partial hematologic responsequalify as CR, and a greater than 50% reduction in the BM MC and serum tryptase level as partial remission. These response criteria were evaluated in the avapritinib phase I EXPLORER trial on a post-hoc basis, showing a high correlation with similar ORR (75% per IWG-MRT-ECNM criteria vs. 77% per PPR criteria). However, there CR and CRh rates were higher with PPR criteria (47%) versus the mIWG-MRT-ECNM criteria (36%). Additionally, there were 11 more patients with AdvSM that were unevaluable by mIWG-MRT-ECNM criteria who were evaluable by PPR criteria.[85,86]

For a complex disease such as AdvSM, a comprehensive response assessment must not only include the histopathologic response, but also the changes in KIT mutant allele, improvement in SM-related organ damage, response of AHN if present, and overall improvement in quality of life. To that effect, a tiered approach encompassing all the above-mentioned parameters is in the making—the ECNM-AIM (The American Initiative in Mast cell diseases) response criteria.[85] Tier IA includes PPR, IB for AHN (if present), Tier II includes *KIT* D816V molecular response, Tier III specifies clinical responses in C-findings, and Tier IV pertains to the quality of life.

The evolution of response criteria in AdvSM over time underscores the complexity and difficulty in capturing different parameters relevant to an objective response to therapy. These newly proposed response criteria still need to be evaluated and validated in prospective clinical trials in the future for AdvSM, and more modifications will likely be required as we generate more knowledge on this complex disease. The hope is the much-needed emphasis on accuracy and objectivity will not defeat practicability.

CONCLUSION AND FUTURE PERSPECTIVES

AdvSM is a heterogenous and complex disease characterized by MC-related organ damage and frequently an associated myeloid malignancy. Over the last few years, significant strides have been made in understanding AdvSM pathogenesis, improving diagnostic accuracy, and developing effective treatments by targeting KIT D816V— the primary oncogenic driver. Midostaurin, a multi-kinase inhibitor, was the first drug approved with significant clinical activity, but the responses were not durable, and tolerability was poor. Avapritinib is a selective KIT D816V inhibitor with much better tolerability that has shown high rates of typically durable responses, achieving a significant reduction in *KIT* D816V allele burden and BM MC. Bezuclastinib and elenestinib are 2 novel potent KIT D816V inhibitors currently undergoing investigation with promising preliminary results. Although these novel KIT inhibitors are very effective against the SM component, their effect on the AHN portion is unclear and given their selectivity for KIT, they are unlikely to be superior to avapritinib in this respect. At this point, AHN treatment relies on AHN-specific therapy, most commonly with hypomethylating agents or AML-type induction chemotherapy. Further studies are needed to explore combination therapies of different AHN treatments with KIT inhibitors. Moreover, modifications to the existing response assessment criteria are needed to make them more practical, objective, and accurate in capturing different dimensions of treatment responses. Additionally, prognostic markers and risk models require re-validation in the KIT inhibitor era. Given the complexity of the diagnosis and treatment of AdvSM, patients should be treated in a multidisciplinary setting at a tertiary referral center with expertise in AdvSM treatment

DISCLOSURE

T. Tashi: Consultant and an investigator for Blueprint Medicines, Cogent Biosciences and PharmaEssentia. M. Deininger: Consultant honorarium and advisory for Blueprint, Novartis, CTIBio Pharma, University of Kansas, GSK Pharma and Ascentage Pharma.

CLINICS CARE POINTS

- SM diagnosis is based on the WHO diagnostic criteria.

- After SM diagnosis is established, mast-cell-related end-organ damage (C-findings) must be assessed, considering that end-organ damage and/or the cytopenias can be due to the SM component or the AHN component, unrelated comorbidities or prior therapies.

- Mediator-release symptoms should be treated with antihistamines, leukotriene inhibitors, mast cell stabilizers and IgE antibodies in a stepwise approach, maximizing the dose of one agent before considering additional agents. Patients often need higher than over-the-counter doses of antihistamines.

- In patients with SM-AHN, clinical determination needs to be made whether to treat SM first or the AHN first or treat both concurrently.

- SM-AHN patients treated with KIT inhibitors should be closely monitored for the acquisition of new somatic mutations and clonal progression. On progression, referral to bone marrow transplant should be made if it is appropriate for the AHN type.

REFERENCES

1. Bibi S, Langenfeld F, Jeanningros S, et al. Molecular defects in mastocytosis: KIT and beyond KIT. Immunol Allergy Clin North Am 2014;34(2):239–62.
2. Furitsu T, Tsujimura T, Tono T, et al. Identification of mutations in the coding sequence of the proto-oncogene c-kit in a human mast cell leukemia cell line causing ligand-independent activation of c-kit product. J Clin Invest 1993; 92(4):1736–44.
3. Helbig G, Koclega A, Gawel WB, et al. The Efficacy of Cladribine (2-CdA) in Advanced Systemic Mastocytosis. Indian J Hematol Blood Transfus 2020;36(4): 661–6.
4. Lim KH, Pardanani A, Butterfield JH, et al. Cytoreductive therapy in 108 adults with systemic mastocytosis: Outcome analysis and response prediction during treatment with interferon-alpha, hydroxyurea, imatinib mesylate or 2-chlorodeoxyadenosine. Am J Hematol 2009;84(12):790–4.
5. DeAngelo DJ, George TI, Linder A, et al. Efficacy and safety of midostaurin in patients with advanced systemic mastocytosis: 10-year median follow-up of a phase II trial. Leukemia 2018;32(2):470–8.

6. Gotlib J, Kluin-Nelemans HC, George TI, et al. Efficacy and Safety of Midostaurin in Advanced Systemic Mastocytosis. N Engl J Med 2016;374(26):2530–41.

7. Lubke J, Schwaab J, Naumann N, et al. Superior Efficacy of Midostaurin Over Cladribine in Advanced Systemic Mastocytosis: A Registry-Based Analysis. J Clin Oncol 2022;40(16):1783–94.

8. Bose P, Verstovsek S. Avapritinib for Systemic Mastocytosis. Expert Rev Hematol 2021;14(8):687–96.

9. Gotlib J, Reiter A, DeAngelo DJ. Avapritinib for advanced systemic mastocytosis. Blood 2022;140(15):1667–73.

10. Gotlib J, Reiter A, Radia DH, et al. Efficacy and safety of avapritinib in advanced systemic mastocytosis: interim analysis of the phase 2 PATHFINDER trial. Nat Med 2021;27(12):2192–9.

11. Reiter A, Gotlib J, Alvarez-Twose I, et al. Efficacy of avapritinib versus best available therapy in the treatment of advanced systemic mastocytosis. Leukemia 2022;36(8):2108–20.

12. Reiter A, Schwaab J, DeAngelo DJ, et al. Efficacy and safety of avapritinib in previously treated patients with advanced systemic mastocytosis. Blood Adv 2022; 6(21):5750–62.

13. Dave N, Devlin M, Rodstrom J, et al. Safety and pharmacokinetics of BLU-263, a next-generation KIT inhibitor. In: Normal healthy volunteers. Abstract. Cancer Res (Supplement); 2021. p. 81. https://doi.org/10.1158/1538-7445.AM2021-CT122.

14. DeAngelo D, Pullarkat VA, Piris-Villaespesa M, et al. Preliminary Safety and Efficacy from Apex, a Phase 2 Study of Bezuclastinib (CGT9486), a Novel, Highly Selective, Potent KIT D816V Tyrosine Kinase Inhibitor, in Adults with Advanced Systemic Mastocytosis (AdvSM). Blood 2022;(140):1.

15. Cruse G, Metcalfe DD, Olivera A. Functional deregulation of KIT: link to mast cell proliferative diseases and other neoplasms. Immunol Allergy Clin North Am 2014; 34(2):219–37.

16. Yuzawa S, Opatowsky Y, Zhang Z, et al. Structural basis for activation of the receptor tyrosine kinase KIT by stem cell factor. Cell 2007;130(2):323–34.

17. Garcia-Montero AC, Jara-Acevedo M, Teodosio C, et al. KIT mutation in mast cells and other bone marrow hematopoietic cell lineages in systemic mast cell disorders: a prospective study of the Spanish Network on Mastocytosis (REMA) in a series of 113 patients. Blood 2006;108(7):2366–72.

18. Sotlar K, Colak S, Bache A, et al. Variable presence of KITD816V in clonal haematological non-mast cell lineage diseases associated with systemic mastocytosis (SM-AHNMD). J Pathol 2010;220(5):586–95.

19. Grootens J, Ungerstedt JS, Ekoff M, et al. Single-cell analysis reveals the KIT D816V mutation in haematopoietic stem and progenitor cells in systemic mastocytosis. EBioMedicine 2019;43:150–8.

20. Jawhar M, Schwaab J, Schnittger S, et al. Molecular profiling of myeloid progenitor cells in multi-mutated advanced systemic mastocytosis identifies KIT D816V as a distinct and late event. Leukemia 2015;29(5):1115–22.

21. Schwaab J, Schnittger S, Sotlar K, et al. Comprehensive mutational profiling in advanced systemic mastocytosis. Blood 2013;122(14):2460–6.

22. Traina F, Visconte V, Jankowska AM, et al. Single nucleotide polymorphism array lesions, TET2, DNMT3A, ASXL1 and CBL mutations are present in systemic mastocytosis. PLoS One 2012;7(8):e43090.

23. Kristensen T, Preiss B, Broesby-Olsen S, et al. Systemic mastocytosis is uncommon in KIT D816V mutation positive core-binding factor acute myeloid leukemia. Leuk Lymphoma 2012;53(7):1338–44.

24. Yin J, Zhu F, Zhang ZB, et al. Rapid and deep response to avapritinib in heavily treated acute myeloid leukemia with t (8;21) and KIT mutation. Ann Hematol 2022; 101(10):2347–50.

25. Pullarkat V, Bedell V, Kim Y, et al. Neoplastic mast cells in systemic mastocytosis associated with t(8;21) acute myeloid leukemia are derived from the leukemic clone. Leuk Res 2007;31(2):261–5.

26. Pullarkat ST, Pullarkat V, Kroft SH, et al. Systemic mastocytosis associated with t(8;21)(q22;q22) acute myeloid leukemia. J Hematop 2009;2(1):27–33.

27. Cornet E, Dumezy F, Roumier C, et al. Involvement of a common progenitor cell in core binding factor acute myeloid leukaemia associated with mastocytosis. Leuk Res 2012;36(11):1330–3.

28. Kim HJ, Ahn HK, Jung CW, et al. KIT D816 mutation associates with adverse outcomes in core binding factor acute myeloid leukemia, especially in the subgroup with RUNX1/RUNX1T1 rearrangement. Ann Hematol 2013;92(2):163–71.

29. Yui S, Kurosawa S, Yamaguchi H, et al. D816 mutation of the KIT gene in core binding factor acute myeloid leukemia is associated with poorer prognosis than other KIT gene mutations. Ann Hematol 2017;96(10):1641–52.

30. Akin C, Fumo G, Yavuz AS, et al. A novel form of mastocytosis associated with a transmembrane c-kit mutation and response to imatinib. Blood 2004;103(8): 3222–5.

31. Bachet JB, Landi B, Laurent-Puig P, et al. Diagnosis, prognosis and treatment of patients with gastrointestinal stromal tumour (GIST) and germline mutation of KIT exon 13. Eur J Cancer 2013;49(11):2531–41.

32. Cammenga J, Horn S, Bergholz U, et al. Extracellular KIT receptor mutants, commonly found in core binding factor AML, are constitutively active and respond to imatinib mesylate. Blood 2005;106(12):3958–61.

33. Hirota S, Isozaki K, Moriyama Y, et al. Gain-of-function mutations of c-kit in human gastrointestinal stromal tumors. Science 1998;279(5350):577–80.

34. Alvarez-Twose I, Gonzalez P, Morgado JM, et al. Complete response after imatinib mesylate therapy in a patient with well-differentiated systemic mastocytosis. J Clin Oncol 2012;30(12):e126–9.

35. Castells M, Butterfield J. Mast Cell Activation Syndrome and Mastocytosis: Initial Treatment Options and Long-Term Management. J Allergy Clin Immunol Pract 2019;7(4):1097–106.

36. Valent P, Sotlar K, Sperr WR, et al. Refined diagnostic criteria and classification of mast cell leukemia (MCL) and myelomastocytic leukemia (MML): a consensus proposal. Ann Oncol 2014;25(9):1691–700.

37. Valent P, Akin C, Metcalfe DD. Mastocytosis: 2016 updated WHO classification and novel emerging treatment concepts. Blood 2017;129(11):1420–7.

38. Arber DA, Orazi A, Hasserjian RP, et al. International Consensus Classification of Myeloid Neoplasms and Acute Leukemias: integrating morphologic, clinical, and genomic data. Blood 2022;140(11):1200–28.

39. Khoury JD, Solary E, Abla O, et al. The 5th edition of the World Health Organization Classification of Haematolymphoid Tumours: Myeloid and Histiocytic/Dendritic Neoplasms. Leukemia 2022;36(7):1703–19.

40. Greiner G, Gurbisz M, Ratzinger F, et al. Digital PCR: A Sensitive and Precise Method for KIT D816V Quantification in Mastocytosis. Clin Chem 2018;64(3): 547–55.

41. Sperr WR, Jordan JH, Fiegl M, et al. Serum tryptase levels in patients with mastocytosis: correlation with mast cell burden and implication for defining the category of disease. Int Arch Allergy Immunol 2002;128(2):136–41.

42. Sperr WR, Kundi M, Alvarez-Twose I, et al. International prognostic scoring system for mastocytosis (IPSM): a retrospective cohort study. Lancet Haematol 2019;6(12):e638–49.

43. Sperr WR, El-Samahi A, Kundi M, et al. Elevated tryptase levels selectively cluster in myeloid neoplasms: a novel diagnostic approach and screen marker in clinical haematology. Eur J Clin Invest 2009;39(10):914–23.

44. Lyons JJ. Hereditary Alpha Tryptasemia: Genotyping and Associated Clinical Features. Immunol Allergy Clin North Am 2018;38(3):483–95.

45. Greiner G, Sprinzl B, Gorska A, et al. Hereditary alpha tryptasemia is a valid genetic biomarker for severe mediator-related symptoms in mastocytosis. Blood 2021;137(2):238–47.

46. Butterfield J, Weiler CR. The Utility of Measuring Urinary Metabolites of Mast Cell Mediators in Systemic Mastocytosis and Mast Cell Activation Syndrome. J Allergy Clin Immunol Pract 2020;8(8):2533–41.

47. Rossini M, Zanotti R, Orsolini G, et al. Prevalence, pathogenesis, and treatment options for mastocytosis-related osteoporosis. Osteoporos Int 2016;27(8): 2411–21.

48. DeAngelo DJ, Radia DH, George TI, et al. Safety and efficacy of avapritinib in advanced systemic mastocytosis: the phase 1 EXPLORER trial. Nat Med 2021; 27(12):2183–91.

49. Pardanani A, Reeder T, Li CY, et al. Eosinophils are derived from the neoplastic clone in patients with systemic mastocytosis and eosinophilia. Leuk Res 2003; 27(10):883–5.

50. Lasho TL, Finke CM, Zblewski D, et al. Novel recurrent mutations in ethanolamine kinase 1 (ETNK1) gene in systemic mastocytosis with eosinophilia and chronic myelomonocytic leukemia. Blood Cancer J 2015;5(1):e275.

51. Gambacorti-Passerini CB, Donadoni C, Parmiani A, et al. Recurrent ETNK1 mutations in atypical chronic myeloid leukemia. Blood 2015;125(3):499–503.

52. Kennedy VE, Perkins C, Reiter A, et al. Mast Cell Leukemia: Clinical and Molecular Features and Survival Outcomes of Patients in the ECNM Registry. Blood Adv 2022. https://doi.org/10.1182/bloodadvances.2022008292.

53. Casassus P, Caillat-Vigneron N, Martin A, et al. Treatment of adult systemic mastocytosis with interferon-alpha: results of a multicentre phase II trial on 20 patients. Br J Haematol 2002;119(4):1090–7.

54. Pardanani A. How I treat patients with indolent and smoldering mastocytosis (rare conditions but difficult to manage). Blood 2013;121(16):3085–94.

55. Barete S, Lortholary O, Damaj G, et al. Long-term efficacy and safety of cladribine (2-CdA) in adult patients with mastocytosis. Blood 2015;126(8):1009–16, quiz 1050.

56. Tefferi A, Kittur J, Farrukh F, et al. Cladribine therapy for advanced and indolent systemic mastocytosis: Mayo Clinic experience in 42 consecutive cases. Br J Haematol 2022;196(4):975–83.

57. Druker BJ, Talpaz M, Resta DJ, et al. Efficacy and safety of a specific inhibitor of the BCR-ABL tyrosine kinase in chronic myeloid leukemia. N Engl J Med 2001; 344(14):1031–7.

58. Deininger MW, Druker BJ. Specific targeted therapy of chronic myelogenous leukemia with imatinib. Pharmacol Rev 2003;55(3):401–23.

59. Vega-Ruiz A, Cortes JE, Sever M, et al. Phase II study of imatinib mesylate as therapy for patients with systemic mastocytosis. Leuk Res 2009;33(11):1481–4.

60. Droogendijk HJ, Kluin-Nelemans HJ, van Doormaal JJ, et al. Imatinib mesylate in the treatment of systemic mastocytosis: a phase II trial. Cancer 2006;107(2): 345–51.

61. Pardanani A, Elliott M, Reeder T, et al. Imatinib for systemic mast-cell disease. Lancet 2003;362(9383):535–6.

62. Ma Y, Zeng S, Metcalfe DD, et al. The c-KIT mutation causing human mastocytosis is resistant to STI571 and other KIT kinase inhibitors; kinases with enzymatic site mutations show different inhibitor sensitivity profiles than wild-type kinases and those with regulatory-type mutations. Blood 2002;99(5):1741–4.

63. Laine E, Chauvot de Beauchene I, Perahia D, et al. Mutation D816V alters the internal structure and dynamics of c-KIT receptor cytoplasmic region: implications for dimerization and activation mechanisms. PLoS Comput Biol 2011;7(6): e1002068.

64. Alvarez-Twose I, Matito A, Morgado JM, et al. Imatinib in systemic mastocytosis: a phase IV clinical trial in patients lacking exon 17 KIT mutations and review of the literature. Oncotarget 2017;8(40):68950–63.

65. Fabbro D, Ruetz S, Bodis S, et al. PKC412–a protein kinase inhibitor with a broad therapeutic potential. Anti Cancer Drug Des 2000;15(1):17–28.

66. Evans EK, Gardino AK, Kim JL, et al. A precision therapy against cancers driven by KIT/PDGFRA mutations. Sci Transl Med 2017;9(414).

67. George S, Jones RL, Bauer S, et al. Avapritinib in Patients With Advanced Gastrointestinal Stromal Tumors Following at Least Three Prior Lines of Therapy. Oncol 2021;26(4):e639–49.

68. DeAngelo D, Reiter A, George T, et al. AZURE: A Phase 1/2 Study of Blu-263 As Monotherapy and in Combination with Azacitidine in Patients with Advanced Systemic Mastocytosis. Abstract. Blood 2022;140:6877–8. ASH Abstract.

69. Guarnieri A, Chicarelli M, Cable L, et al. Preclinical Data with KIT D816V Inhibitor Bezuclastinib (CGT9486) Demonstrates High Selectivity and Minimal Brain Penetrance. Abstract. Blood 2021;(138):1.

70. Gotlib J, Baird JH, George TI, et al. A phase 2 study of brentuximab vedotin in patients with CD30-positive advanced systemic mastocytosis. Blood Adv 2019; 3(15):2264–71.

71. Jawhar M, Schwaab J, Naumann N, et al. Response and progression on midostaurin in advanced systemic mastocytosis: KIT D816V and other molecular markers. Blood 2017;130(2):137–45.

72. Deininger M, DeAngelo D, Radia D, et al. Effective Control of Advance Systemic Mastocytosis with Avapritinib: Mutational Analysis from the Explorer Clinical Study. Abstract. Blood 2021;(138):1. https://doi.org/10.1182/blood-2021-150872.

73. Lim KH, Wu JN, Huang TY, et al. Clonal evolution and heterogeneity in advanced systemic mastocytosis revealed by single-cell DNA sequencing. Blood Adv 2021; 5(6):1733–6.

74. Reiter A, George TI, Gotlib J. New developments in diagnosis, prognostication, and treatment of advanced systemic mastocytosis. Blood 2020;135(16):1365–76.

75. Ustun C, Reiter A, Scott BL, et al. Hematopoietic stem-cell transplantation for advanced systemic mastocytosis. J Clin Oncol 2014;32(29):3264–74.

76. Ustun C, Gotlib J, Popat U, et al. Consensus Opinion on Allogeneic Hematopoietic Cell Transplantation in Advanced Systemic Mastocytosis. Biol Blood Marrow Transplant 2016;22(8):1348–56.

77. Lim KH, Tefferi A, Lasho TL, et al. Systemic mastocytosis in 342 consecutive adults: survival studies and prognostic factors. Blood 2009;113(23):5727–36.

78. Pardanani A, Lim KH, Lasho TL, et al. Prognostically relevant breakdown of 123 patients with systemic mastocytosis associated with other myeloid malignancies. Blood 2009;114(18):3769–72.
79. Jawhar M, Schwaab J, Schnittger S, et al. Additional mutations in SRSF2, ASXL1 and/or RUNX1 identify a high-risk group of patients with KIT D816V(+) advanced systemic mastocytosis. Leukemia 2016;30(1):136–43.
80. Munoz-Gonzalez JI, Jara-Acevedo M, Alvarez-Twose I, et al. Impact of somatic and germline mutations on the outcome of systemic mastocytosis. Blood Adv 2018;2(21):2814–28.
81. Jawhar M, Schwaab J, Alvarez-Twose I, et al. MARS: Mutation-Adjusted Risk Score for Advanced Systemic Mastocytosis. J Clin Oncol 2019;37(31):2846–56.
82. Pardanani A, Shah S, Mannelli F, et al. Mayo alliance prognostic system for mastocytosis: clinical and hybrid clinical-molecular models. Blood Adv 2018;2(21):2964–72.
83. Gotlib J, Pardanani A, Akin C, et al. International Working Group-Myeloproliferative Neoplasms Research and Treatment (IWG-MRT) & European Competence Network on Mastocytosis (ECNM) consensus response criteria in advanced systemic mastocytosis. Blood 2013;121(13):2393–401.
84. Valent P, Akin C, Sperr WR, et al. Aggressive systemic mastocytosis and related mast cell disorders: current treatment options and proposed response criteria. Leuk Res 2003;27(7):635–41.
85. Gotlib J, Schwaab J, Shomali W, et al. Proposed European Competence Network on Mastocytosis-American Initiative in Mast Cell Diseases (ECNM-AIM) Response Criteria in Advanced Systemic Mastocytosis. J Allergy Clin Immunol Pract 2022;10(8):2025–2038 e1.
86. Shomali W, Gotlib J. Response Criteria in Advanced Systemic Mastocytosis: Evolution in the Era of KIT Inhibitors. Int J Mol Sci 2021;22(6). https://doi.org/10.3390/ijms22062983.

Tyrosine Kinase Inhibitors in Non-advanced Systemic Mastocytosis

Cem Akin, MD, PhD

KEYWORDS

- Mastocytosis • KIT D816V mutation • Tyrosine kinase inhibitors • Avapritinib
- Imatinib • Midostaurin

KEY POINTS

- Systemic mastocytosis is driven by KIT D816V mutation in more than 90% of the cases. KIT D816V is a gain of function mutation resulting in intrinsic tyrosine kinase activity of KIT without requiring ligand binding.
- Tyrosine kinase inhibitors with inhibitory activity against D816V KIT have been approved for advanced systemic mastocytosis. Recently avapritinib gained approval as the first such TKI for treatment of indolent SM.
- Tyrosine kinase inhibitors have been shown to reduce neoplastic mast cells and improve symptoms in clinical trials of advanced and non-advanced SM.
- Mutational status of KIT D816V should be checked by a highly sensitive technique such as allele-specific PCR or digital droplet PCR before the consideration of a targeted therapy.

INTRODUCTION

Non-advanced systemic mastocytosis (SM) makes up the majority of cases among patients with systemic mastocytosis.[1] Features of non-advanced SM include the absence of other clonal hematologic (myeloid) disorders, or tissue dysfunction attributable to mast cell infiltration, low rate of progression to advanced disease, and a life expectancy which is comparable to age-matched general population. Non-advanced SM consists of 3 distinct subcategories: Indolent systemic mastocytosis constitutes the majority of patients.[1] Bone marrow mastocytosis defines a group of patients with low mast cell burden (tryptase < 125 ng/mL) and no skin lesions, and smoldering systemic mastocytosis with high mast cell burden (tryptase levels >200 ng/mL, or bone marrow mast cell infiltrate of >30%, dysmyelopoiesis without an overt associated non-mast cell myeloid clonal disease, and organomegaly without tissue dysfunction).[2]

Division of Allergy and Clinical Immunology, Department of Internal Medicine, University of Michigan, 24 Frank Lloyd Wright Drive, PO Box 442, Suite H-2100, Ann Arbor, MI 48106-0442, USA
E-mail address: cemakin@umich.edu

Immunol Allergy Clin N Am 43 (2023) 743–750
https://doi.org/10.1016/j.iac.2023.05.001
0889-8561/23/© 2023 Elsevier Inc. All rights reserved.
immunology.theclinics.com

Mortality related to disease progression or complications is rare in non-advanced SM.[3] However, there is no curative option for the disease and a subset of patients still experience reduced quality of life and are in need of new therapeutic options. The first line of treatment in non-advanced SM is antimediator therapy, variably combining H1 and H2 histamine receptor antagonists, anti-leukotriene agents, and mast cell stabilizers such as cromolyn sodium.[4] Patient symptomatology show a considerable variation. While some patients are minimally symptomatic and only need occasional as needed H1 antihistamine therapy for symptoms such as flushing and itching, others may experience recurrent epsidoes of mast cell activation with additional symptoms including abdominal pain, diarrhea, tachycardia, and vascular instability and chronic symptoms such as memory changes, and musculoskeletal pain, despite being on multiple antimediator medications.[5]

TYROSINE KINASE INHIBITORS IN NON-ADVANCED SYSTEMIC MASTOCYTOSIS

The rationale for tyrosine kinase inhibition (TKI) therapy of SM lies in the fact that the majority (>90%) of patients with SM carry the D816V somatic gain of function mutation in the receptor tyrosine kinase KIT.[6,7] This mutation confers ligand (stem cell factor) independent activation of KIT which causes mast cell growth, differentiation and protection from apoptosis. KIT is also involved in mast cell activation pathways and its stimulation is thought to reduce the activation threshold of mast cells, leading to mediator-related symptoms. KIT D816V mutation is expressed in both advanced and non-advanced SM. However, in patients with non-advanced mastocytosis, the mutation is generally restricted to the mast cell lineage while patients with advanced variants display the mutation in multiple cell linages[8] and also carry mutations such as *ASXL1, RUNX1, TET2 and SRSF2* in other hematopoietic genes.[9] Demonstration that KIT D816V inhibitors caused reductions in neoplastic mast cell numbers along with partial and complete disease remissions, and improved survival in advanced mastocytosis (reviewed elsewhere in this volume) led to FDA approval of these agents for advanced mastocytosis. Therefore, this positive experience in advanced disease lead to consideration of non-advanced disease even a more attractive target for these drugs as the KIT D816V mutation is generally the only molecular defect demonstrated in these patients.

KIT TKIs can be divided into 3 main groups. (1). Those inhibit only wild-type (WT) KIT or non-codon D816V mutations (eg, imatinib), (2). TKIs that inhibit both WT and D816V KIT mutants (eg, midostaurin), and (3). Selective KIT D816V inhibitors (eg, avapritinib, elenestinib, bezuclastinib).[10] Imatinib is the prototypical TKI which inhibits WT KIT along with ABL, FLT3, PDGFRA, PDGFRB, and CSFR1. It was the first TKI approved to treat advanced mastocytosis without KIT D816V mutation or unknown KIT mutation status. The initial approval of this drug for SM was influenced by the positive effect of the drug on patients with chronic eosinophilic leukemia or myeloproliferative variant hypereosinophilic syndrome characterized by PDGFRA rearrangements, which is a molecular target for imatinib.[11] In addition to a profound eosinophilia, these patients have some overlapping criteria for mastocytosis including morphologically atypical increased mast cells which express CD25, and a modest elevation in serum tryptase levels, although the disease pathology is manifested due to eosinophilia and not mastocytosis.[12] Rare patients, mostly belonging to the histopathologic subvariant of well differentiated mastocytosis may have a WT KIT or non-codon D816V mutations responsive to imatinib.[13] For example, the first demonstration of response to TKI therapy was reported in a patient with F522C transmembrane KIT mutation who responded to imatinib.[14] Before contemplating therapy with imatinib due to a negative KIT D816V test, it should be ascertained that the method of detection of the mutation has a high level of sensitivity (such as allele specific PCR or didgital droplet PCR), capable of detecting an allele burden of 0.1% or lower.[15] Mutation detection assays based on sequencing such as next generation sequencing panels lack the sensitivity to detect a low burden mutation which is the case for most patients with bone marrow mastocytosis or ISM. Therefore, imatinib is not an option for the great majority of patients with SM who carry the D816V mutation and is not approved for non-advanced mastocytosis.

Midostaurin is a multi-kinase inhibitor with activity against both WT and D816V KIT.[16] It also inhibits IgE-mediated mast cell activation.[17] It has been approved for advanced mastocytosis based on a Phase 2 open-label study on 116 patients with advanced SM, which showed an overall response rate of 60% and reductions in bone marrow mast cell burden.[18] Patients in this study were also shown to have significant improvements in quality of life measures.[19] The most common side effect was gastrointestinal toxicity, with nausea, vomiting and diarrhea occurring in 79%, 66% and 54% of the patients. Grade 3 to 4 hematologic toxicity and cytopenias were also seen in 24% to 41% of the patients, most of whom had preexisting cytopenias. In an open-label trial of midostaurin in 20 patients with ISM, 38% reduction in symptom severity was observed at 24 months.[20] Recent retrospective chart review data from Mayo Clinic experience with midostaurin in 13 patients with non-advanced SM showed similar efficacy data and high rate of dose reduction (75%) due to side effects.[21] Overall, midostaurin is not indicated for non-advanced disease and its utility is limited by its gastrointestinal toxicity.

Avapritinib is a D816V selective KIT inhibitor, currently approved for the treatment of advanced and indolent SM. Approval for advanced SM was based on EXPLORER and PATHFINDER studies on 131 patients with advanced disease who achieved an overall response rate of 75%, with improvement in mast cell-related tissue damage, and reductions in bone marrow mast cell burden, tryptase and KIT D816V variant allele fraction.[22–24] Major side effects included periocular and peripheral edema, diarrhea, and nausea (50, 23, 18% respectively). Intracranial bleeding occurred in 9 patients (13%) in EXPLORER trial, and 8 of them were associated with thrombocytopenia of less than 50×10^9/L. Cognitive dysfunction, mostly grades 1 to 2, was observed in 11% of the patients. PIONEER study evaluated avapritinib in ISM. After a dose finding first part of the study, 25 mg daily dose was selected as the part 2 dose (as compared to 200 mg starting daily dose in advanced mastocytosis).[25] In part 2 of the PIONEER study, 212 patients with ISM were randomized to receive avapritinib versus placebo.[26,27] The primary outcome was change in a composite score based on 11 symptoms at 24 weeks of treatment, which was significantly improved in patients receiving avapritinib as compared to placebo. Improvements in key secondary endpoints included reductions in serum tryptase, bone marrow mast cell infiltration and KIT D816V variant allele fraction. In addition, avapritinib significantly improved skin lesions, improved the quality of life and reduced polypharmacy. The drug was well tolerated with peripheral and periorbital edema being the side effects (6.8% each) observed more frequently than placebo (1.4% and 2.8% respectively). Cognitive adverse events were similar in avapritinib (2.8%) versus placebo (4.2%), and there were no intracranial bleeds. Overall, these results indicate that avapritib was safe and effective in this patient population. Based on these results, avapritinib was approved by FDA on May 22, 2023 for the indication of indolent systemic mastocytosis.[28]

Elenestinib (BLU-263) and bezuclastinib are investigational KIT D816V selective inhibitors that have similar potency to avapritinib in KIT D816V inhibition but with minimal brain penetration as compared to avapritinib.[29–32] In addition, bezuclastinib has been reported to lack significant inhibitory activity against structurally related kinases PDGFRA, PDGFRB, FLT3, CSFR1.[33] Both drugs are in clinical trials in non-advanced

Table 1
Selected KIT tyrosine kinase inhibitors and their status in non-advanced SM

Drug	KIT Inhibition	Approval in SM	Current Clinical Trials in Non-Advanced SM (clinicaltrials.gov Identifier)	Additional Notes
Imatinib	WT	Approved for advanced SM without KIT D816V mutation or unknown mutation status	-	Not an effective option for the majority of patients who carry D816V mutation.
Midostaurin	WT and D816V	Approved for advanced SM	-	Use in non-advanced disease limited by gastrointestinal toxicity
Avapritinib	D816V	Approved for advanced and indolent SM.	PIONEER (NCT03731260)	Favorable efficacy and safety profile in PIONEER trial
Elenestinib	D816V	Investigational	HARBOR (NCT04910685)	Does not have CNS penetration
Bezuclastinib	D816V	Investigational	SUMMIT (NCT05186753)	Does not have CNS penetration, lacks significant inhibitory activity against PDGFR, CSF1R, FLT3

mastocytosis (**Table 1**). These clinical trials employ a similar methodology and design as the PIONEER trial, consisting of a dose finding part, followed by an expansion phase of the selected dose versus placebo and a long-term follow-up phase after unblinding and roll over of placebo patients to active treatment.

Anaphylaxis is one of the most feared symptoms in SM, occurring in up to 50% of adult patients.[34] Preliminary reports suggest that TKIs may be effective in reducing or preventing anaphylaxis in patients with SM;[19,35] however, patient numbers are limited and more studies are needed to explore whether TKIs may be of benefit in the prophylaxis of anaphylaxis in SM. KIT D816V specific TKIs can theoretically reduce the potential for anaphylaxis by reducing mast cell numbers in tissues and around blood vessels and by inhibiting the additive activation potential in IgE and non–IgE-mediated mast cell activation pathways. To that end, it remains to be explored how susceptibility to anaphylaxis correlates with mast cell cytoreduction, and whether TKIs could be used for a limited time or as premedications in patients with hymenoptera venom allergies or part of desensitization protocols in patients with SM, who could not tolerate these protocols otherwise.[36] In addition, the efficacy of TKIs in monoclonal mast cell activation syndrome (MMAS, a clonal disease variant characterized by recurrent mast cell activation symptoms and detection of KIT D816V variant allele in low frequencies but not fully meeting the diagnostic criteria for mastocytosis) remains to be explored. To that end, clinical trial with elenestinib includes a cohort of patients with MMAS.

SUMMARY AND FUTURE PERSPECTIVES

The selection of patients for TKI therapy should involve a shared decision making considering the benefits and risks of these therapies.[10] It is likely that these drugs will be needed as long term or indefinite treatment. Clinical trials of TKIs in non-advanced disease included patients who remain symptomatic despite being on at least 2 anti-mediator therapy options (or intolerant of them due to side effects), and such patients are the obvious candidates for these novel drugs. Patients with prior history of intracranial bleeding and thrombocytopenia should be excluded from therapy with avapritinib. The benefits of improvements in disease symptoms, skin lesions, quality of life, reduction in polypharmacy, and avoiding the side effects of antimediator drugs should be weighed against the unknown potential long-term side effects, the possibility of reproductive toxicity in a demographic population of patients who include those in their childbearing ages.

Future research on TKI therapy of mastocytosis is needed to answer critical questions. In addition to questions pertaining to anaphylaxis above, it remains to be seen how co-morbidities such as osteoporosis, venom allergy and hard to treat symptoms such musculosleletal pain, brain fog, and fatigue will respond to long term TKI treatment. Patients with non-advanced SM can have a wide spectrum of mast burden ranging from low burden bone marrow mastocytosis to high-burden smoldering systemic mastocytosis, and it is not clear whether a single dose would be similarly effective in all of these categories. The optimum duration of therapy, the effects of TKIs on disease progression, and the role of combination therapies with non-TKI drugs are also among questions to be explored.

CLINICS CARE POINTS

- Avapritinib, a TKI with selective inhibitory profile of D816 V mutated as compared to wild type KIT, has been shown to be effective in reducing symptom severity and mast cell burden in Phase 2 clinical trial (PIONEER), and became the first TKI to be approved by FDA for treatment of indolent SM.

- Clinical trials with other selective D816V KIT inhibitors (elenestinib and bezuclastinib) are currently in progress.
- Detection of D816 V KIT mutation patients with non-advanced disease should be done by a highly sensitive method such as allele-specific PCR or digital droplet PCR instead of next-generation sequencing panels which may lack sensitivity to detect a low-level mutated allele burden. Testing of lesional tissue such as bone marrow is preferrable.

CONFLICT OF INTEREST STATEMENT

Dr C. Akin receives research support from Blueprint Medicines and Cogent Biosciences, and has consultancy agreements with Blueprint, Cogent and Novartis.

REFERENCES

1. Valent P, Oude Elberink JNG, Gorska A, et al. Study Group of the European Competence Network on Mastocytosis (ECNM). The Data Registry of the European Competence Network on Mastocytosis (ECNM): Set Up, Projects, and Perspectives. J Allergy Clin Immunol Pract 2019;7(1):81–7.
2. Valent P, Akin C, Hartmann K, et al. Updated Diagnostic Criteria and Classification of Mast Cell Disorders: A Consensus Proposal. Hemasphere 2021;5(11): e646.
3. Trizuljak J, Sperr WR, Nekvindová L, et al. Clinical features and survival of patients with indolent systemic mastocytosis defined by the updated WHO classification. Allergy 2020;75(8):1927–38.
4. Valent P, Hartmann K, Schwaab J, et al. Personalized Management Strategies in Mast Cell Disorders: ECNM-AIM User's Guide for Daily Clinical Practice. J Allergy Clin Immunol Pract 2022;10(8):1999–2012.e6.
5. Mesa RA, Sullivan EM, Dubinski D, et al. Patient-reported outcomes among patients with systemic mastocytosis in routine clinical practice: Results of the Touch-Stone SM Patient Survey. Cancer 2022;128(20):3691–9.
6. Akin C, Metcalfe DD. The biology of Kit in disease and the application of pharmacogenetics. J Allergy Clin Immunol 2004;114(1):13–9, quiz 20.
7. Bibi S, Langenfeld F, Jeanningros S, et al. Molecular defects in mastocytosis: KIT and beyond KIT. Immunol Allergy Clin North Am 2014;34(2):239–62.
8. Garcia-Montero AC, Jara-Acevedo M, Teodosio C, et al. KIT mutation in mast cells and other bone marrow hematopoietic cell lineages in systemic mast cell disorders: a prospective study of the Spanish Network on Mastocytosis (REMA) in a series of 113 patients. Blood 2006;108(7):2366–72.
9. Schwaab J, Schnittger S, Sotlar K, et al. Comprehensive mutational profiling in advanced systemic mastocytosis. Blood 2013 Oct 3;122(14):2460–6.
10. Akin C, Arock M, Valent P. Tyrosine kinase inhibitors for the treatment of indolent systemic mastocytosis: Are we there yet? J Allergy Clin Immunol 2022;149(6): 1912–8.
11. Pardanani A, Ketterling RP, Brockman SR, et al. CHIC2 deletion, a surrogate for FIP1L1-PDGFRA fusion, occurs in systemic mastocytosis associated with eosinophilia and predicts response to imatinib mesylate therapy. Blood 2003;102(9): 3093–6.

12. Maric I, Robyn J, Metcalfe DD, et al. KIT D816V-associated systemic mastocytosis with eosinophilia and FIP1L1/PDGFRA-associated chronic eosinophilic leukemia are distinct entities. J Allergy Clin Immunol 2007;120(3):680–7.

13. Alvarez-Twose I, Matito A, Morgado JM, et al. Imatinib in systemic mastocytosis: a phase IV clinical trial in patients lacking exon 17 *KIT*mutations and review of the literature. Oncotarget 2016;8(40):68950–63.

14. Akin C, Fumo G, Yavuz AS, et al. A novel form of mastocytosis associated with a transmembrane c-kit mutation and response to imatinib. Blood 2004;103(8): 3222–5.

15. Hoermann G, Sotlar K, Jawhar M, et al. Standards of Genetic Testing in the Diagnosis and Prognostication of Systemic Mastocytosis in 2022: Recommendations of the EU-US Cooperative Group. J Allergy Clin Immunol Pract 2022;10(8): 1953–63.

16. Growney JD, Clark JJ, Adelsperger J, et al. Activation mutations of human c-KIT resistant to imatinib mesylate are sensitive to the tyrosine kinase inhibitor PKC412. Blood 2005;106(2):721–4.

17. Krauth MT, Mirkina I, Herrmann H, et al. Midostaurin (PKC412) inhibits immunoglobulin E-dependent activation and mediator release in human blood basophils and mast cells. Clin Exp Allergy 2009;39(11):1711–20.

18. Gotlib J, Kluin-Nelemans HC, George TI, et al. Efficacy and Safety of Midostaurin in Advanced Systemic Mastocytosis. N Engl J Med 2016;374(26):2530–41.

19. Hartmann K, Gotlib J, Akin C, et al. Midostaurin improves quality of life and mediator-related symptoms in advanced systemic mastocytosis. J Allergy Clin Immunol 2020;146(2):356–66.e4.

20. van Anrooij B, Oude Elberink JNG, Span LFR, et al. Midostaurin in patients with indolent systemic mastocytosis: An open-label phase 2 trial. J Allergy Clin Immunol 2018;142(3):1006–8.e7.

21. Farrukh F, Gangat N, Shah MV, et al. Midostaurin therapy for indolent and smoldering systemic mastocytosis: Retrospective review of Mayo Clinic experience. Am J Hematol 2022;97(4):E138–40.

22. DeAngelo DJ, Radia DH, George TI, et al. Safety and efficacy of avapritinib in advanced systemic mastocytosis: the phase 1 EXPLORER trial. Nat Med 2021; 27(12):2183–91.

23. Gotlib J, Reiter A, Radia DH, et al. Efficacy and safety of avapritinib in advanced systemic mastocytosis: interim analysis of the phase 2 PATHFINDER trial. Nat Med 2021;27(12):2192–9.

24. Castells M, Akin C. Finding the right KIT inhibitor for advanced systemic mastocytosis. Nat Med 2021;27(12):2081–2.

25. Akin, Cem et al. PIONEER: A Randomized, Double-Blind, Placebo-Controlled, Phase 2 Study of Avapritinib in Patients with Indolent or Smoldering Systemic Mastocytosis (SM) With Symptoms Inadequately Controlled by Standard Therapy. Journal of Allergy and Clinical Immunology, Volume 145, Issue 2, AB336.

26. Castells, Mariana et al., Efficacy and Safety of Avapritinib in Indolent Systemic Mastocytosis (ISM): Results from the Double Blinded Placebo-Controlled PIONEER Study Journal of Allergy and Clinical Immunology, Volume 151, Issue 2, AB204.

27. www.blueprintmedicines.com/wp-content/uploads/2023/02/Blueprint-Medicines-AAAAI-2023-Avapritinib-Indolent-SM-PIONEER-Efficacy-Safety-Oral-Presentation. pdf. Accessed May 15, 2023.

28. Gotlib J, Castells M, Elberin HO, et al. Avapritinib versus placebo in indolent systemic mastocytosis. New Engl J Med Evid 2023;2(6). https://doi.org/10.1056/EVIDoa2200339.

29. Gotlib J. Available and emerging therapies for bona fide advanced systemic mastocytosis and primary eosinophilic neoplasms. Hematology Am Soc Hematol Educ Program 2022;2022(1):34–46.

30. Castells M, Bhavsar V, He K, Scherber R, Akin C. HARBOR, a phase 2/3 study of BLU-263 in patients with indolent systemic mastocytosis and monoclonal mast cell activation syndrome abstract. Paper presented at: European Hematology Association Congress; 10 June 2022; Vienna, Austria.

31. www.blueprintmedicines.com/wp-content/uploads/2022/02/Blueprint-Medicines-AAAAI-2022-HARBOR-BLU-263-Indolent-Systemic-Mastocytosis.pdf Accessed May 15, 2023.

32. Akin C. Summit: A 3-Part, Phase 2 Study of Bezuclastinib (CGT9486), an Oral, Selective, and Potent KIT D816V Inhibitor, in Adult Patients with Nonadvanced Systemic Mastocytosis (NonAdvSM). ASH; 2022 cited 2023 Mar 14. Available from: https://ash.confex.com/ash/2022/webprogram/Paper156326.html.

33. www.cogentbio.com/wp-content/uploads/2022/12/ASH-2022-Summit-TiP.pdf Accessed May 15, 2023.

34. Brockow K, Jofer C, Behrendt H, et al. Anaphylaxis in patients with mastocytosis: a study on history, clinical features and risk factors in 120 patients. Allergy 2008; 63(2):226–32.

35. Kudlaty E, Perez M, Stein BL, et al. Systemic mastocytosis with an associated hematologic neoplasm complicated by recurrent anaphylaxis: Prompt resolution of anaphylaxis with the addition of avapritinib. J Allergy Clin Immunol Pract 2021; 9(6):2534–6.

36. Castells MC, Hornick JL, Akin C. Anaphylaxis after hymenoptera sting: is it venom allergy, a clonal disorder, or both? J Allergy Clin Immunol Pract 2015;3(3):350–5.

Measuring Symptom Severity and Quality of Life in Mastocytosis

Polina Pyatilova, MD[a,b], Frank Siebenhaar, MD[a,b],*

KEYWORDS

- Mastocytosis • Symptoms • Signs • Quality of life • Assessment • Disease burden

KEY POINTS

- Mastocytosis is a heterogeneous disorder with variable clinical course and phenotypes.
- Several disease-related signs and symptoms are nonspecific for mastocytosis, including anaphylaxis, osteoporosis, cardiovascular, gastrointestinal, and neurocognitive symptoms, and their associated underlying cause remains largely unknown.
- Difficult-to-diagnose phenotypes (ie, absence of skin involvement, bone marrow mastocytosis) are less well characterized in terms of symptom profiles and treatment responses.
- Patients with CM and non-AdvSM are mostly affected by mast cell mediator–related symptoms, whereas in AdvSM symptoms also result from organ damage, which makes their assessment challenging.

INTRODUCTION

Mastocytosis is a complex group of disorders with a variable course and heterogenous clinical phenotypes, ranging from asymptomatic to highly severe.[1,2] Because of a multiorgan involvement, patients are cared for by specialists from many fields, including dermatology, hematology, allergology/clinical immunology, internal medicine, and neurology.[3,4] Skin lesions, anaphylaxis, osteoporosis, gastrointestinal (GI) involvement, and organomegaly may be present or not. Guided by the leading sign, symptom, or affected organ, various diagnostic measures and tools are used to evaluate patients' disease and symptom burden. Although significant advances have been made in defining and diagnosing the burden of disease, assessing symptom burden remains a challenge. The ideal tools to address this challenge should (1) be disease-specific and cover all spectra of mastocytosis, (2) be easy to use and able

[a] Institute of Allergology, Charité - Universitätsmedizin Berlin, Corporate Member of Freie Universität Berlin and Humboldt-Universität zu Berlin, Berlin, Germany; [b] Fraunhofer Institute for Translational Medicine and Pharmacology, Immunology and Allergology, Berlin, Germany
* Corresponding author. Charité - Universitätsmedizin Berlin, Institute of Allergology, Hindenburgdamm 30, Paul-Ehrlich-Haus, Berlin 12203, Germany.
E-mail address: frank.siebenhaar@charite.de

Immunol Allergy Clin N Am 43 (2023) 751–762
https://doi.org/10.1016/j.iac.2023.04.003   immunology.theclinics.com
0889-8561/23/© 2023 Elsevier Inc. All rights reserved.

to assess and monitor symptom burden in everyday life and in clinical trials, and (3) allow comparison of outcomes between patients with different clinical phenotypes.

MASTOCYTOSIS PHENOTYPES

Patients with mastocytosis differ regarding disease prognosis, being classified as having indolent forms of mastocytosis, including cutaneous mastocytosis, indolent systemic mastocytosis (ISM), and smoldering systemic mastocytosis; or advanced forms of systemic mastocytosis (AdvSM), such as aggressive systemic mastocytosis, systemic mastocytosis with an associated myeloid neoplasm, or mast cell leukemia.

AdvSM presents with cytopenia, hepatomegaly accompanied by impaired liver function and ascites, splenomegaly with hypersplenism, malabsorption, weight loss, and/or large osteolytic lesions. Organ damage and its consequences are the main findings in AdvSM. Patients with AdvSM have a less favorable prognosis and should be monitored and cared for by hematologic specialists.

ISM is diagnosed more frequently, in about 90% of adult patients with mastocytosis. In contrast to AdvSM, patients with ISM have a good prognosis and normal survival, but are at risk to exhibit skin lesions and to experience mast cell mediator–related symptoms. The analysis of the patient registry of the European Competence Network on Mastocytosis in 2021 revealed that cutaneous involvement strongly correlates with disease subtypes and is almost always present in ISM, in most smoldering systemic mastocytosis, and in less than half of aggressive systemic mastocytosis and mast cell leukemia cases.[5] However, it is a common observation that existing subgroups of patients may predispose for specific combinations of signs and symptoms and thereby represent distinguished clinical phenotypes. For example, patients with ISM without skin involvement are at higher risk for anaphylactic reactions.[6,7] **Fig. 1** highlights more than 20 possible combinations of disease-related signs and symptoms, which could be present in patients with mastocytosis. To our current knowledge, most patients present with skin lesions (>80%), whereas osteopenia/osteoporosis and anaphylaxis are diagnosed in about 10% to 20% of patients.[8] Typical skin involvement, characterized by the evidence of maculopapular red-brown lesions accompanied in most cases by Darier sign, remains the most robust and specific clinical sign of mastocytosis. Patients without skin lesions are diagnosed less frequently, in most cases because of an anaphylactic reaction in medical history[9] but rarely caused by isolated osteoporosis, GI symptoms, or neurocognitive complaints. However, the percentage of patients with and without skin involvement, anaphylaxis, osteoporosis, and GI tract involvement, varies widely between studies, emphasizing the potential heterogeneity in patient populations or diagnostic approaches used. Anaphylaxis is difficult to assess in the medical history and may be easily confused with syncope of other nature because predictors and long-term biomarkers are lacking. Finally, for some frequently reported symptoms, such as fatigue, headache, brain fog, cognitive disorders, palpitations, weakness, dizziness, and pain in different regions of the body, mastocytosis-related pathogenesis and disease-specificity are poorly defined. As a result, defining distinct clinical phenotypes in mastocytosis seems to be challenging, because the presence of multiple disease-related signs and symptoms is influenced by nonspecific and/or secondary signs and symptoms, which in turn may lead to inconsistent treatment responses and blurred outcome measures. Such nonspecific or secondary signs and symptoms may occur because of a concomitant disorder or side effects to current therapy. Taken together, stratifying patients into distinct clinical phenotypes requires that (1) all disease-specific symptoms are defined; (2) established criteria and analysis of impact for each symptom exists; and (3) disease

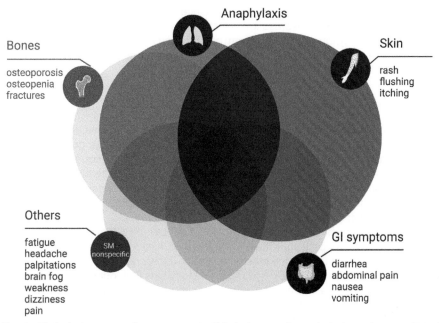

Fig. 1. Clinical phenotypes in mastocytosis. Skin lesions and anaphylaxis are known clinical signs of mastocytosis, followed by bone involvement (ie, osteoporosis/osteopenia/spontaneous fractures) and gastrointestinal complains. The cohorts are visualized based on an expert opinion and are not supported statistically.

management is concise, resulting in standardized diagnosis and assessment of signs and symptoms in patients with mastocytosis.

DISEASE BURDEN FROM A PATIENT PERSPECTIVE

Patients with AdvSM suffer from organ damage, which, in early stages, is difficult to quantify and monitor. It should be considered that some GI symptoms, such as abdominal pain and vomiting, could be provoked by organomegaly and reflect a severe course of disease. Most bothersome symptoms in AdvSM are GI and skin symptoms. Vomiting, diarrhea, and nausea could also be drug-related.[10]

In contrast, patients with ISM are not affected by organ damage but may suffer from various signs and symptoms, which could be severe and tremendously impair quality of life (QoL). Cutaneous, GI, and skeletal symptoms are the most common complaints in mastocytosis. When analyzing a large cohort, 70% of mostly patients with ISM reported to feeling disabled because of the disease-associated symptoms.[11] Psychological and neurologic symptoms markedly influence the feeling of disability, and the psychological impact of cutaneous signs and symptoms, fatigue, and itch ranked among the top three complaints.[11] However, it is largely unknown whether neuropsychological symptoms are disease-mediated or rather associated with a concomitant disorder or potentially related to a current therapy.

ISM significantly affects QoL, relationships within the family, and social communications.[12,13] Patients must restrict several activities because of a high symptom burden. Psychological and physical symptoms affect QoL in mastocytosis,[13] with the fear of an anaphylaxis being one of the main factors impacting patients' QoL.[11,14,15] Longer symptom duration and high need for therapy was also shown to be associated with

QoL impairment.[16] A third of patients experience anxiety and about 10% to 15% report being depressed or express low satisfaction with life.[15] The relative impact of disease-specific symptoms or symptom combinations and respective complaints caused by a potential concomitant disorder on QoL impairment has not been clearly defined and should be addressed in future studies.

HOW TO ASSESS SYMPTOM SEVERITY AND QUALITY OF LIFE

According to the consensus opinion of the European and American experts involved in the management of mastocytosis, the following validated four-score grading system has been introduced in 2007, where 0 is no symptoms; 1 is mild, infrequent, no therapy required; 2 is mild/moderate, frequent, kept under control with therapy; 3 is severe, frequent, difficult to control; and 4 is severe adverse event/hospitalization required, with further frequency evaluation, being A for less than 1 episode per year, B for 1 to 12 episodes per year, and C for greater than 1 per month.[17]

Since then several patient-reported outcome measures (PROMs) have been developed and validated for patients with indolent forms of mastocytosis: the mastocytosis symptom assessment form[14]; the mastocytosis activity score (MAS)[18]; the ISM symptom assessment form (ISM-SAF)[19]; and the mastocytosis QoL questionnaires developed and validated in a German (MC-QoL),[20] Dutch (MQLQ),[14] and Polish (QLMS)[15] cohort of patients (Table 1). A separate tool for symptom assessment in AdvSM, the AdvSM symptom assessment form, has been introduced in 2021.[19] Recall periods, details on items and domains, and scoring systems are summarized in Table 1.

Results of the AFFIRM score[11] were presented in 2008 on a large cohort of patients with mastocytosis. It is a complex questionnaire, which includes 38 symptoms and covers 12 areas: skin, allergy/flush/shock, GI tract, rheumatology, asthenia, neurology/psychiatry, respiratory, urology, infection, hemorrhoidal inflammation, libido, and sweating. The items were generated based on the results of patient interviews. For each symptom the grade and impact on the QoL impairment are asked.

The mastocytosis symptom assessment form was first developed to assess symptom severity in mastocytosis, and underwent item generation, item reduction, and validation. It resulted in a shorter symptom assessment form, consisting of 14 items. Moreover, it includes an additional domain with five questions on the impact of fatigue on everyday life with a recall on the last 24 hours.[14]

The MAS, validated in 2018, focuses on nine main symptoms that resulted from item generation by semistructured patient interviews and subsequent impact analysis.[18] Total score and domain scores of each of the three domains (ie, skin, GI tract, and other symptoms) could be extracted. This gives an opportunity to identify not only the total disease burden but different phenotypes separately. To obtain robust data, it is recommended to be completed daily for 14 consecutive days.

ISM-SAF and AdvSM are the latest symptom assessment forms, developed and sponsored by industry, and are currently used in ongoing clinical trials.[19,21,22] The ISM-SAF can be applied to patients with cutaneous mastocytosis and ISM, whereas the AdvSM symptom assessment form was designed and validated for AdvSM. The ISM-SAF consists of 12 items and is easy to complete. This PROM for the first time includes "spots" and "diarrhea frequency" in the set of questions. Similar to the MAS, a total score and domain scores for skin and GI domains can be assessed.

Three disease-specific QoL tools are currently available for patients with indolent forms of mastocytosis. They assess QoL impairment retrospectively, evaluating the impact of disease aspects over 2 weeks, which makes it much easier to be used in everyday clinical practice. The MC-QoL consists of 27 questions each with a

Table 1
Available approaches to assess symptom severity and QoL impairment in patients with mastocytosis

	PROM/Score	Completion	Items/Domains	Parameter	Grade Definition
CM/ISM Symptoms	ECNM-AIM criteria EU/US Consensus 2007	—	—	Skin and MC-mediated symptoms	0–4, where 0: no 1: mild, infrequent, no therapy required 2: mild/moderate, frequent, control with therapy 3: severe, frequent, difficult to control 4: severe adverse event/hospitalization required (4A, <1 episode/year; 4B, 1–12 episodes/y; 4C, >1/mo)
	AFFIRM France 2008	—	38 items/12 domains	Skin, allergy/flush/shock, GI, rheumatology, asthenia, neurology/psychiatry, respiratory, urology, infection, hemorrhoidal inflammation, libido, sweat	0: none 1: light 2: moderate 3: severe 4: intolerable + Impact of the symptom on QoL (1–5)
	MSAF[a] Netherlands 2016	—	14 items	Itching, flushing, dizziness, headache, fatigue, mediator-release attacks, dyspnea, rhinorrhea, palpitations, nausea and vomiting, abdominal pain, bone pain, concentration problems, depression	0–10, where 0: absent 10: very severe
		Recall period 24 h	1 additional domain	Influence of fatigue	0–10, where 0: no influence 10: maximum influence

(continued on next page)

Table 1
(continued)

PROM/Score	Completion	Items/Domains	Parameter	Grade Definition
MAS[a] Germany 2018	7–14 consecutive days	9 items	Itching, skin redness/swelling, flushing, diarrhea, abdominal cramping, muscle/joint pain, fatigue/exhaustion, headache, difficulty concentrating	0–4, where 0: not at all 1: mild 2: moderate 3: severe 4: very severe
		3 domains	Skin, GI, and other	
ISM-SAF[a,b] 2021	7–14 consecutive days	12 items		Spots, itching, flushing, diarrhea, abdominal pain, nausea, bone pain, fatigue, dizziness, brain fog, headache, diarrhea frequency
2 domains Skin and GI		0–10, where 0: no 10: worst imaginable		
QoL				
MC-QoL[a] Germany 2016	Once, recall period 2 wk	27 items/4 domains	Symptoms, emotions, social life/functioning, and skin	0–4, where 0: none 1: somewhat 2: moderately 3: very 4: very much
MQLQ[a] Netherlands 2016	Once	49 items/8 domains	Fatigue and mental health, anaphylaxis, bone symptoms, unfamiliarity (low awareness), flushing, general symptoms, skin symptoms, and triggers	0–6, where 0: none, or not applicable 1: hardly 2: somewhat 3: moderately 4: considerably 5: severely 6: worst possible
QLMS[a] Poland 2021	Once	24 items/4 domains	Leisure time, protective behaviors, professional life and life	0–5, where 0: no 5: prevent normal functioning

| AdvSM | Symptoms | AdvSM-SAF[a,b] 2021 | 7 consecutive days | 10 items | Spots, itching, flushing, diarrhea, abdominal pain, vomit, nausea, fatigue, vomit frequency, diarrhea frequency | 0–10, where 0: no 10: worst imaginable |
| | | | | 2 domains | Skin and GI | |

Abbreviations: AdvSM-SAF, advanced systemic mastocytosis symptom assessment form; CM, cutaneous mastocytosis; ECNM, European Competence Network on Mastocytosis; ISM-SAF, indolent systemic mastocytosis symptom assessment form; MC, mast cell; MSAF, mastocytosis symptom assessment form.

[a] Underwent item generation, item selection, and final validation.
[b] Developed by industry (Adelphi Values and Blueprint Medicines).

five-point Likert scale and four domains on symptoms, emotions, social life/functioning, and skin.[20] The MQLQ has 49 items and eight domains (ie, fatigue and mental health, anaphylaxis, bone symptoms, unfamiliarity [low awareness], flushing, general symptoms, skin symptoms, and triggers).[14] Differently from the MC-QoL and the QLMS, it includes more questions on the role of different symptoms on QoL impairment. The recently developed QLMS is the most compact PROM for QoL assessment.[15] It is the first tool that takes avoidance strategies and protective behaviors of patients into account, because they are at risk of experiencing anaphylaxis. It could be of great benefit to be used in patients with mastocytosis, especially in those who had previously severe anaphylactic reactions.

DISCUSSION

Do the Available Patient-Reported Outcome Measures Cover the Right and Relevant Signs and Symptoms in Mastocytosis?

No effective drugs that show good symptom reduction in patients with indolent forms of mastocytosis are currently available. This fact makes it even more difficult to identify the true cause of disease-related symptoms, particularly neurocognitive complaints that many patients suffer from, and how they are associated with mastocytosis. For example, a clinical study with the anti-Siglec-8 antibody lirentelimab (AK002) showed better response of GI and skin symptoms as compared with fatigue and concentration difficulty.[23] A French study showed that patients with mastocytosis suffer from at least 32 symptoms with a significantly higher prevalence when compared with healthy control subjects.[11] The biggest challenge in designing a scoring PROM is how to keep it short and effective but also applicable and comprehensive for such a complex disease as mastocytosis. The current disease-specific PROMs are aimed to cover the most important aspects of the disease, stay short, and cover the symptoms known to be linked to the disease. Because knowledge in the field of mastocytosis in terms of diagnostic procedures that resulted in a more advanced classification and risk stratification for disease progression has incredibly increased over the past years, it is still challenging to come up with the ideal approach to assess symptom burden and QoL impairment by PROMs because the characterization and definition of distinct disease phenotypes is still under investigation. Today, an increasing number of patients are diagnosed in an early stage of their disease, which makes it even more important to define and differentiate the disease-specific symptomatology in these novel phenotypes of mastocytosis from complaints that could be associated with another concomitant and/or preexisting disorder. For example, patients without mastocytosis in the skin (MIS) are now getting diagnosed more frequently because of increased awareness and access to highly sensitive genetic evaluation for the KIT D816V mutation. This gives the opportunity to diagnose patients without MIS, in which other predominant signs and symptoms, such as anaphylaxis, osteoporosis, pain, GI symptoms, and others, led to a suspicion of mastocytosis. However, this advantage is accompanied by a potential clinical dilemma. For example, there are several limitations to identify GI manifestations in mastocytosis because robust histologic findings are lacking to clearly link them to disease pathogenesis. In fact, a debilitating GI manifestation is reported by more than half of patients with mastocytosis, but it is nonspecific and therefore difficult to distinguish from other chronic GI disorders, such as irritable bowel syndrome.[24,25] Several mastocytosis-specific PROMs have been designed and translated to multiple languages, making them accessible around the world.[11,14,18,19] The future use of these tools in larger patient cohorts, the way they perform in the setting of clinical trials, and their capability to document clinical response to targeted treatments will finally result in a better understanding of the symptomatology associated with mastocytosis and its different phenotypes.

Do the Available Patient-Reported Outcome Measures Correctly Reflect the Quality of Life Impairment in All Patients with Mastocytosis?

Health-related QoL in mastocytosis has been previously investigated and shown to significantly impact QoL by using disease-specific tools.[13–15,20] Whereas each of these tools provide robust and valid data, there are yet no studies that compare the outcomes of different available PROMs in the same cohort of patients. Moreover, it is largely unknown whether patients with different clinical presentations also exhibit different levels of QoL impairment and what is the major driver of QoL impairment associated with distinct clinical phenotypes. For example, do patients where the predominant symptom is itch experience a similar or higher discomfort than patients suffering from GI symptoms or vice versa? To answer this question PROMs would need to be developed and validated in patients with different prevalent symptoms (ie, with distinct clinical phenotypes) separately. The results of a Dutch study in a large cohort of patients with ISM showed no association between the prevalence of MIS, osteoporosis, or anaphylaxis and the level of QoL impairment, suggesting that QoL is independent of a certain predominant sign/symptom.[14] Of note, patients that experienced previous episodes of anaphylaxis have been reported to express a high level of anxiety and experience drastic restrictions to their everyday life, which significantly affects QoL.[14,15] Yet, it remains to be investigated how different levels of QoL impairment would translate to different clinical phenotypes irrespective of the tool being used. The tools currently available are extensively designed to include virtually all aspects of the disease and have been validated in mixed patient populations, with the risk that actual differential impacts of the disease on QoL may go undetected because of mathematical bias. Thus, further studies performed in stratified patient populations with distinct clinical phenotypes are needed to identify the impact of different disease aspects on the level of QoL impairment.

How to Better Evaluate Signs/Symptoms and Quality of Life in Mastocytosis?

As mentioned previously, there is a variety of PROMs available for the assessment of symptom severity and QoL. Comparative studies between different tools are lacking, which makes it impossible to link the scores achieved by different PROMs to each other. Harmonization is desirable and could be achieved by using a single tool to be applied in all patients and clinical studies or normalizing the scores from different tools to make them comparable.

The cause of nonspecific symptoms, including fatigue, brain fog, palpitations, headache, and others, need to be better investigated and classified to identify and differentiate between disease-specific, treatment-related, and concomitant symptoms and to finally define distinct clinical phenotypes.

Unmet Needs

- Identification and definition of distinct clinical disease phenotypes.
- Evaluation of symptom specificity by analyzing the performance of PROMs on targeted treatment of patients with indolent forms of mastocytosis.
- Better characterization of the symptomatology of patients without skin involvement (MIS).
- Harmonization of the results assessed by different existing disease-specific PROMs.

- Investigation of the impact of different symptoms and symptom combinations on the level of QoL impairment.

SUMMARY

The fact that many different factors influence the impact of disease on a patient perspective becomes a specific matter of interest because these factors are expected to respond differently to targeted treatment strategies. The definition of clinical phenotypes and better characterization of the respective factors that influence the impact and patient perspective on symptom burden and QoL impairment is yet an unmet need that requires further investigation in future health care–related studies in mastocytosis.

CLINICS CARE POINTS

- When measuring disease burden, identify disease-related signs and symptoms, including anaphylaxis, osteopenia/osteoporosis, and skin involvement, and cutaneous, gastrointestinal, and musculoskeletal symptoms.
- Fatigue, headache, brain fog, cognitive disorders, palpitations, weakness, dizziness, and pain in different regions of the body should be assessed with caution, because their pathogenesis and disease specificity are poorly defined.
- To assess symptom severity use currently available PROMs, validated for patients with indolent or advanced forms of mastocytosis.
- Quality of life is frequently impaired in patients with mastocytosis and should be assessed in all patients by using disease-specific tools (ie, MC-QoL, MQLQ, or QLMS).

CONFLICTS OF INTEREST

P. Pyatilova has no relevant conflict of interest in relation to this work. F. Siebenhaar is or recently was a speaker and/or advisor for and/or has received research funding from Allakos, Blueprint, Celldex, Cogent, Escient, Granular, GSK, Invea, Novartis, Moxie, Sanofi/Regeneron, Third Harmonic, and Uriach.

REFERENCES

1. Valent P, Akin C, Sperr WR, et al. New insights into the pathogenesis of mastocytosis: emerging concepts in diagnosis and therapy. Annu Rev Pathol 2023;18: 361–86.
2. Valent P, Akin C, Hartmann K, et al. Updated diagnostic criteria and classification of mast cell disorders: a consensus proposal. Hemasphere 2021;5(11):e646.
3. Broesby-Olsen S, Dybedal I, Gulen T, et al. Multidisciplinary management of mastocytosis: Nordic Expert Group Consensus. Acta Derm Venereol 2016;96(5):602–12.
4. Valent P, Akin C, Gleixner KV, et al. Multidisciplinary challenges in mastocytosis and how to address with personalized medicine approaches. Int J Mol Sci 2019;20(12). https://doi.org/10.3390/ijms20122976.
5. Aberer E, Sperr WR, Bretterklieber A, et al. Clinical impact of skin lesions in mastocytosis: a multicenter study of the European Competence Network on Mastocytosis. J Invest Dermatol 2021;141(7):1719–27.
6. Gulen T, Ljung C, Nilsson G, et al. Risk factor analysis of anaphylactic reactions in patients with systemic mastocytosis. J Allergy Clin Immunol Pract 2017;5(5): 1248–55.

7. Alvarez-Twose I, Zanotti R, Gonzalez-de-Olano D, et al. Nonaggressive systemic mastocytosis (SM) without skin lesions associated with insect-induced anaphylaxis shows unique features versus other indolent SM. J Allergy Clin Immunol 2014;133(2):520–8.

8. Valent P, Hartmann K, Schwaab J, et al. Personalized management strategies in mast cell disorders: ECNM-AIM user's guide for daily clinical practice. J Allergy Clin Immunol Pract 2022;10(8):1999–2012 e6.

9. Pardanani A, Tefferi A. Systemic mastocytosis in adults: a review on prognosis and treatment based on 342 Mayo Clinic patients and current literature. Curr Opin Hematol 2010;17(2):125–32.

10. Shomali W, Gotlib J. Response criteria in advanced systemic mastocytosis: evolution in the era of KIT inhibitors. Int J Mol Sci 2021;(6):22. https://doi.org/10.3390/ijms22062983.

11. Hermine O, Lortholary O, Leventhal PS, et al. Case-control cohort study of patients' perceptions of disability in mastocytosis. PLoS One 2008;3(5):e2266.

12. Jensen B, Broesby-Olsen S, Bindslev-Jensen C, et al. Everyday life and mastocytosis from a patient perspective-a qualitative study. J Clin Nurs 2019;28(7–8):1114–24.

13. Vermeiren MR, Kranenburg LW, van Daele PLA, et al. Psychological functioning and quality of life in patients with mastocytosis: a cross-sectional study. Ann Allergy Asthma Immunol 2020;124(4):373–378 e2.

14. van Anrooij B, Kluin-Nelemans JC, Safy M, et al. Patient-reported disease-specific quality-of-life and symptom severity in systemic mastocytosis. Allergy 2016;71(11):1585–93.

15. Spolak-Bobryk N, Niedoszytko M, Jassem E, et al. The role of the clinical and psychological symptoms of mastocytosis in the patient's quality of life. Postepy Dermatol Alergol 2022;39(4):688–96.

16. Pulfer S, Ziehfreund S, Gebhard J, et al. Health-related quality of life and influencing factors in adults with nonadvanced mastocytosis: a cross-sectional study and qualitative approach. J Allergy Clin Immunol Pract 2021;9(8):3166–3175 e2.

17. Valent P, Akin C, Escribano L, et al. Standards and standardization in mastocytosis: consensus statements on diagnostics, treatment recommendations and response criteria. Eur J Clin Invest 2007;37(6):435–53.

18. Siebenhaar F, Sander B, Ho LHT, et al. Development and validation of the mastocytosis activity score. Allergy 2018;73(7):1489–96.

19. Taylor F, Akin C, Lamoureux RE, et al. Development of symptom-focused outcome measures for advanced and indolent systemic mastocytosis: the AdvSM-SAF and ISM-SAF((c)). Orphanet J Rare Dis 2021;16(1):414.

20. Siebenhaar F, von Tschirnhaus E, Hartmann K, et al. Development and validation of the mastocytosis quality of life questionnaire: MC-QoL. Allergy 2016;71(6):869–77.

21. Taylor F, Li X, Yip C, et al. Psychometric evaluation of the Advanced Systemic Mastocytosis Symptom Assessment Form (AdvSM-SAF). Leuk Res 2021;108:106606.

22. Padilla B, Shields AL, Taylor F, et al. Psychometric evaluation of the Indolent Systemic Mastocytosis Symptom Assessment Form (ISM-SAF) in a phase 2 clinical study. Orphanet J Rare Dis 2021;16(1):434.

23. Siebenhaar F, Bonnekoh H, Hawro T, et al. Safety and efficacy data of AK002, an anti-siglec-8 monoclonal antibody, in patients with indolent systemic mastocytosis (ISM): Results from a first-in-human, open-label phase 1 study. Abstracts LB TPS. Allergy 2019;74(S106):910–1.

24. Zanelli M, Pizzi M, Sanguedolce F, et al. Gastrointestinal manifestations in systemic mastocytosis: the need of a multidisciplinary approach. Cancers 2021; 13(13).
25. Sokol H, Georgin-Lavialle S, Canioni D, et al. Gastrointestinal manifestations in mastocytosis: a study of 83 patients. J Allergy Clin Immunol 2013;132(4): 866–873 e1, 3.

Effect of Gender and Special Considerations for Women in Mastocytosis and Anaphylaxis

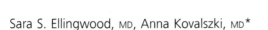

Sara S. Ellingwood, MD, Anna Kovalszki, MD*

KEYWORDS

- Anaphylaxis • Mastocytosis • Sex hormones • Pregnancy • Gender considerations

KEY POINTS

- Incidence of anaphylaxis is increased in female compared with male patients in the pubertal years, but this disparity narrows afterthe age of 55 years.
- Sex hormones are implicated in rare causes of anaphylaxis, such as catamenial, progestogen, and lactation anaphylaxis.
- Estrogen worsens passive anaphylaxis in mouse models by increasing tissue expression of endothelial nitric oxide synthase, which increases vascular permeability.
- Indolent systemic mastocytosis does not appear to affect fertility or pregnancy outcomes but should be managed by a multidisciplinary team with a focus on symptom prevention while minimizing risk to the fetus both during pregnancy and at delivery.
- Incidence of systemic mastocytosis is increased in female patients; however, disease progression and overall survival are significantly worse in male patients owing to increased cytogenetic and molecular abnormalities.

INTRODUCTION

Anaphylaxis is a serious, potentially fatal generalized or systemic hypersensitivity reaction, which is typically rapid in onset and usually characterized by involvement of at least 2 different organ systems (skin, respiratory, cardiovascular, or gastrointestinal). Many clinical studies show the incidence of systemic anaphylaxis differs with respect to gender.[1] The literature suggests that adult women have more frequent anaphylaxis induced by food,[2,3] radiocontrast agents,[4,5] drugs,[6,7] and vaccines[8,9] when compared with adult men. Idiopathic anaphylaxis is also more commonly reported in adult women.[10] Since these differences are present in reproductive years, not prepubertal years, sex hormones appear to play a role in susceptibility to anaphylaxis.[11] Catamenial (or cyclical) anaphylaxis, characterized by recurrent anaphylaxis

Division of Allergy and Clinical Immunology, University of Michigan, 24 Frank Lloyd Wright Drive, Suite H-2100, Ann Arbor, MI, 48106, USA
* Corresponding author.
E-mail address: vidadi@med.umich.edu

Immunol Allergy Clin N Am 43 (2023) 763–776
https://doi.org/10.1016/j.iac.2023.04.004
0889-8561/23/© 2023 Elsevier Inc. All rights reserved.

around the time of menstruation, suggests progesterone or prostaglandins (PGs) may be associated with susceptibility to anaphylaxis.[11,12] Progesterone-associated anaphylaxis and lactation-associated anaphylaxis are also described, which demonstrate the temporal association between the fluctuations of endogenous or exogenous hormones and anaphylaxis in some women.[13] Pregnancy can have a variable influence on immediate hypersensitivity reactions,[6] and consensus guidelines on diagnosis and management of anaphylaxis during pregnancy remain lacking.[14]

ANAPHYLAXIS
Hormonal Pathophysiologic Influences on Anaphylaxis

Hormonal influences on anaphylaxis remain poorly understood. Mouse models assist in understanding the mechanistic basis of the sex bias that is seen between males and females (**Table 1**). Mast cells (MC) are known to have sex hormone receptors, but the receptor triggered component's potential role in anaphylaxis is not known. Recent studies have given insights into potential mechanisms underlying the disparity between anaphylaxis severity in female mice compared with male mice. Hox and colleagues[11] found that estrogen plays a role in potentiation and increased severity of anaphylaxis. This study induced passive anaphylaxis in female and male mice by histamine, immunoglobulin E (IgE), or IgG receptor aggregation. Anaphylactic responses were monitored and found to be more pronounced in female than male mice. Pretreatment with an estrogen receptor antagonist or ovariectomy eliminated the enhanced severity of anaphylaxis. However, increased severity in anaphylaxis was restored after administration of estradiol in ovariectomized mice. In terms of potential mechanism, estrogen was found to increase tissue expression of endothelial nitric oxide synthase (eNOS), which increases vascular permeability. Use of an NOS inhibitor or genetic eNOS deficiency eliminated sex-related differences in anaphylaxis. When anaphylaxis was induced either by a bolus of histamine or by cross-linking FcγRIIIA with 2.4G2, anaphylaxis models that do not require MC activation, anaphylactic reactions were found to be more severe in sham-operated mice compared with ovariectomized mice, suggesting estrogen-mediated potentiation of anaphylaxis is downstream of MC activation and occurs regardless of trigger. Interestingly, estrogen was not found to increase MC responsiveness, suggesting the threshold for anaphylaxis was not changed, however the severity was, and this conflicts with prior studies.[15]

In vitro female primary bone marrow–derived mast cells (BMMCs) have been found to exhibit increased degranulation as they synthesize and store larger amounts of granule mediators (β-hexosaminidase, tumor necrosis factor-α, tryptase, and histamine) than male BMMCs. This has also been seen in female peritoneal MCs and in different animal species, such as mice and rats. Increased degranulation response in female BMMCs results from upregulated expression of a variety of genes, such as tumor necrosis factor (Tnf), phos-phoribosyl pyrophosphate synthetase 1(Prps), Spermidine synthetase (Srm), and Basic helix-loop-helix family member A15 (Bhlha15), involved in metabolic, biosynthetic, and cellular processes leading to MC granule formation.[16,17]

Progesterone is an important metabolic intermediate and has many roles in a spectrum of organ systems, including preparing the uterus for implantation, decreasing the maternal immune response allowing for pregnancy, decreasing uterine smooth muscle contractility, inhibition of lactation during pregnancy, anti-inflammatory effects, and assistance in regulation of T-lymphocyte–mediated immune responses. Progesterone hypersensitivity results in anaphylaxis at the peak of progesterone levels during the luteal phase of the menstruation cycle (see **Table 1**). The mechanism for

Table 1
Effect of sex hormones on anaphylaxis

Hormone	Experimental Models	Ref.	Humans	Ref.
Estrogen	↑Severity of passive anaphylaxis through increased vascular permeability	11	ER expressed by MCs	48
	↑eNOS activity and production in female MCs	11	↑β-Hexosaminidase release in HMC	15
	ERα expressed by MCs and BMMCs	11,15,48	↑Tryptase expression in HMC-1	48
	↑Histamine release in female pMCs	17		
	↑Degranulation and LTC4 production	15		
Progesterone	↓Histamine release in pMCs (rat)	18	↑Tryptase expression in HMC	48
			Catamenial anaphylaxis	12
Prolactin	Unknown		Lactation or breastfeeding anaphylaxis	35,37,38
Androgens	↑Histamine release in female pMCs but not in men by testosterone and DHT (rat)	66	AR expressed by skin MCs	20,21
			↓IL-6 production in female breast skin MC by DHT	20,21

Abbreviations: AR, androgen receptor; DHT, dihydrotestosterone; ER, estrogen receptor; HMC, human mast cells; IL-6, interleukin-6; LTC4, leukotriene C4; MCs, mast cells; pMCs, peritoneal mast cells.

From Salvati L, Vitiello G, Parronchi P. Gender differences in anaphylaxis. Curr Opin Allergy Clin Immunol. 2019;19(5):417-424.

sensitization to progesterone has not been well-defined. Prior studies suggested that progesterone may inhibit histamine secretion from purified rat peritoneal MCs stimulated immunologically or by substance P.[18] Whereas, Zierau and colleagues[19] demonstrated that treatment of human MC lines in vitro with physiologic concentrations ofestradiol and progesterone resulted in significantly increased release of MC β-tryptase.

Androgen receptors are present primarily on skin MCs but have not been found to exert a direct influence on IgE-dependent MC degranulation.[20] Androgens have been found to cause reduced production of interleukin-6 (IL-6) in female breast skin MCs compared with male foreskin MCs. IL-6 has important functions, imparting protection from sepsis and tumor growth, but also contributes to obesity and male-patterned baldness.[21]

The Epidemiology of Anaphylaxis by Trigger

Food allergy

Adolescent boys are more likely to be diagnosed with atopic conditions, including eczema, asthma, and food allergy.[22] Beyond 15 years of age, women are more likely to be diagnosed with both severe food allergy and anaphylaxis. A ratio as high as 60:40 female-to-male predominance of food allergy and anaphylaxis is reported.[22] On the other hand, a review of food-dependent exercise-induced urticaria/angioedema and anaphylaxis showed a slight male predominance (55.4%).[23] Interestingly, the sex disparity in food allergy along with many other allergic triggers diminishes after the fifth decade of life.[24] Daily and lifetime hormonal changes are thought to result in sex-dependent humoral and cellular immune responses that differ among genders. However, the effects of these fluctuations on food allergy diagnosis as well as symptom severity need to be evaluated in future gender-differentiating studies.[24]

Drug anaphylaxis

The female predominance of anaphylaxis is true in many types of drug allergy. A recent review of hypersensitivity reactions to iodinated contrast media (ICM) in Italy showed an increased risk of hypersensitivity reactions owing to female sex and age less than 65 years.[4] A 6-year study of all patients referred to a university hospital in France for suspected ICM allergy evaluated the utility of ICM skin testing. Two-thirds of the patients recruited were women. Interestingly, the male-to-female ratio of those with positive ICM skin prick testing (SPT) was 1:1, and 90% of these participants had immediate reactions. Negative SPT was more common in women with a ratio of 1:2.4, with 70% of participants with immediate reactions. When considering immediate and nonimmediate reactions, the ratio of male to female was 1:1.14 to 1:4.5. This finding was consistent with prior studies that women have increased incidence of hypersensitivity reactions to ICM, and female gender is a risk factor for nonimmediate reactions.[5]

The COVID-19 pandemic and vaccination effort and associated increased scrutiny on reported hypersensitivity reactions also highlight a female predominance of vaccine-associated anaphylactic and nonanaphylactic reactions in multiple studies.[8,9] This trend is appreciated in most other vaccines, particularly in women of childbearing age.[25] A review of vaccine-associated hypersensitivity found the rate of vaccine anaphylaxis to be 1.45 per million vaccine doses in women, compared with 1.14 per million vaccine doses in men.[25] The most commonly implicated vaccines included influenza, Tdap, and varicella.[25]

A recent review of the U.S. Food and Drug Administration Adverse Event Reporting System revealed 15,506,002 drug-related adverse events reported from 1999 to 2019.

Of those adverse events, 47,496 (0.27%) were reported as anaphylaxis. The median age of patients in reports of anaphylaxis was 52 years, and 62.71% were women.[26] Antibiotics were the most common drug class implicated in anaphylactic reactions followed by monoclonal antibodies (MoAb), nonsteroidal anti-inflammatory drugs (NSAIDs) and acetaminophen, and intraoperative agents.[26] Cancer drug anaphylaxis (chemotherapies and MoAb) is recognized as a worldwide complication impacting the quality of life and survival of patients. Platinum-based antineoplastic drugs, taxanes, and MoAbs are most commonly involved. Desensitization protocols have been developed to help mitigate the impact for those who tolerate this mechanism of therapy. Data from centers performing these desensitizations showed that 91% of protocols are performed in women (mean age, 57 years), mainly affected by ovarian cancer, and treated with carboplatin and paclitaxel.[27] It is estimated that 27% of women with ovarian or breast cancer develop carboplatin allergy after several cycles of treatment.[28] Patients who present with BRCA 1 or 2 mutations may be at increased risk for earlier hypersensitivity reactions and reactions during rapid drug desensitization to carboplatin.[29]

Hymenoptera venom anaphylaxis
Along with food and drug allergy, Hymenoptera venom allergy is one of the top 3 causes of anaphylaxis worldwide. Although women are often found to have an increased incidence of anaphylaxis to many other triggers, male sex is an independent risk factor for severe allergic reactions to Hymenoptera venom. The effect of male sex as a risk factor in venom-allergic patients, however, has been mainly attributed to a higher degree of exposure to stinging insects.[30]

Progestogen hypersensitivity
Progestogen hypersensitivity (PH), previously deemed autoimmune progesterone dermatitis, is a heterogenous disorder characterized by hypersensitivity symptoms, including dermatologic (eg, urticaria, angioedema, eczematous dermatitis, petechiae/purpura) and nondermatologic symptoms, such as asthma and anaphylaxis. Symptoms are typically cyclical and occur during the peak progesterone levels of the luteal phase, 3 to 10 days before menstruation, and dissipate a few days into menses. PH is a rare and poorly recognized disorder with unknown prevalence and incidence. The frequency with which anaphylaxis occurs is also not well-defined. PH typically only affects women; however, there is one documented case of hypersensitivity to megestrol acetate in a man confirmed by positive skin testing to progesterone acetate.[31] It is unclear how patients become sensitized to progestogens. One theory is that sensitization occurs with exposure to exogenous progesterone or synthetic progestins used for contraception or hormonal supplementation. Many cases have been associated with supratherapeutic doses of progesterone used for fertility treatments.[13] However, cases exist when there has been no previous exposure to exogenous progestogen.[32] Treatment varies widely based on symptoms and long-term goals, but generally focuses on symptom management and anovulation, if appropriate.[13] Desensitization may also be considered when continuous use of progesterone is needed.[13]

Catamenial anaphylaxis
Catamenial anaphylaxis is also associated with the menstrual cycle; however, timing differs from PH. Symptoms of catamenial anaphylaxis correlate with the onset of the menstrual cycle, which starts with a rapid decline of estrogen and progesterone rather than the peak of progesterone associated with PH. The underlying mechanism of catamenial anaphylaxis is unknown. It has been proposed to be triggered by the

endometrial release of PGs, which are highest on day 1 of the menstrual cycle.[12,13,33] Prostaglandin F2 is synthesized by the endometrium and is related to mediator release by uterine MCs. Differentiating catamenial anaphylaxis from PH is important, as different treatment options are proposed for each condition. Burstein and colleagues[34] reported a patient with recurrent anaphylaxis occurring in the first 24 hours after onset of menses, who had improvement of symptoms after treatment with indomethacin, which inhibits PGs. Complete resolution of symptoms occurred with hysterectomy and salpingo-oophorectomy. Other treatments with variable success include antihistamines, GnRH analogues,[33] corticosteroids, combined oral contraceptives, and omalizumab.[12]

Lactation-associated anaphylaxis

Anaphylaxis associated with lactation is a very rare condition, and reporting is often limited to case reports.[13,35–37] In many cases, the symptoms, ranging from urticaria to hypotension andsyncope, start the first few days after delivery during the act of breastfeeding or with expression of breast milk. Documented elevations in tryptase have been reported.[13,35,36] Anaphylaxis associated with lactation is often experienced with subsequent pregnancies.[36,37] The underlying mechanism of anaphylactic events associated with lactation is not understood. It has been proposed that the rapid decrease in progesterone in the postpartum period may lead to an exaggerated histamine response.[13] Sensitization to hormones associated with lactation, such as prolactin and oxytocin, has been considered, but skin testing has not elicited positive results.[37,38] NSAIDs, which are often used in the postpartum period, have also been thought to be the cause of these anaphylactic events.[13,36,37] Some patients also have eventual resolution of symptoms after a few days of breastfeeding.[37] Some patients have had improvement in symptoms with prophylactic antihistamine use. However, when symptoms remain refractory, suppression of lactation may become necessary.[35,38]

Idiopathic Anaphylaxis

The precise prevalence of idiopathic anaphylaxis is unknown. It remains a diagnosis of exclusion. Multiple studies have found the overall incidence is higher in women compared with men.[10,39] One theory for female predominance from puberty until menopause is that female hormones may exert an unknown effect on MCs.[10,39]

Fatal Anaphylaxis

Although anaphylaxis is a relatively common event, affecting up to 5% of US citizens, fatal anaphylaxis is rare, with a mortality rate less than 1 death per million people per year.[40] Data available from epidemiologic studies exhibit critical limitations in reporting of anaphylaxis owing to numerous factors, including accessibility to care, nonspecific coding, limitations in the electronic medical record reporting, changes of the definition of anaphylaxis over time, lack of confirmatory testing, and selection bias.[16] When considering all causes of anaphylaxis, incidence of anaphylaxis is often found to be higher in women.[2–8] However, male gender appears to be a risk factor for severe anaphylaxis along with higher age, and concomitant mastocytosis. Despite this, many studies show no significant gender differences in all-cause anaphylaxis-associated fatalities.[16,41,42] Gender has not been shown consistently to be an independent risk factor for fatal drug-induced anaphylaxis.[40–42] Drug-induced anaphylaxis followed by death is very rare overall, 2984/17,506,022 (0.01%).[16] The median age of patients reported to have drug-associated anaphylaxis death was 60 years, and

50.19% were women, which highlights the narrowed disparity between female and male anaphylaxis-associated death.[26]

However, a few key disparities have been found when considering fatal anaphylaxis.[16,40–42] Men have a significantly increased risk for fatal anaphylaxis to venom, and African American men have an increased risk for fatal anaphylaxis to foods.[41,42] Unspecified fatal anaphylaxis is significantly associated with older age and African American race.[42]

MASTOCYTOSIS

Mastocytosis is a rare disease that results from a clonal, neoplastic proliferation of morphologically and immunophenotypically abnormal MCs that accumulate in one or more organ systems. The clinical presentation is heterogenous, ranging from skin-limited disease (cutaneous mastocytosis, CM), to bone marrow–involved indolent systemic mastocytosis (ISM), to a more aggressive variant with extracutaneous multi-organ involvement (aggressive systemic mastocytosis), which may be associated with shortened survival.[43] An epidemiologic study in Denmark revealed the prevalence of ISM was higher in women than in men.[44] However, ISM without skin lesions and associated with Hymenoptera venom anaphylaxis (HVA) has a significant male predominance.[45,46] Very rare mast cell leukemia (MCL) is also more common in men.[44] Other subtypes of systemic mastocytosis were found to be slightly more common in women.[44] Most types of systemic mastocytosis (SM) are usually diagnosed in middle age (mean age, 46–61 years); however, MCL is diagnosed later in life (mean age, 75 years).[44]

Presentation of mastocytosis can be variable, ranging from MC mediator and skin symptoms to vasodilatory symptoms. Anaphylaxis is often the presenting symptom in patients with ISM and monoclonal mast cell activation syndrome (MMAS). It is estimated that up to 5% of patients who present with anaphylaxis may have underlying primary MC identifiable activation disorders. The most common cause of anaphylaxis related to ISM is insect sting/bite, followed by idiopathic causes, whereas the most common causes of anaphylaxis in the general population are food and drugs.[45]

Mast Cells in Reproduction and Pregnancy

MCs play a key role in inflammatory reactions owing to allergic and nonallergic processes. The most common trigger for MC degranulation is cross-linking of the high-affinity IgE receptors during immediate hypersensitivity reactions. Other triggers include aggregated IgG, complement proteins, peptides, and sex hormones, which are involved in MC regulation and activation.[47]

MCs are present in the endometrium in all stages of the menstrual cycle, and migration of MC to the uterus in the first stages of pregnancy is regulated by estradiol and progesterone changes.[47,48] Studies are conflicting on the physiologic and pathogenic role of MCs during pregnancy.[49] MC density has been documented to be significantly higher in the myometrium of pregnant women.[47] MC mediators, such as histamine, are found to be essential to pregnancy and delivery, including implantation of the blastocyst, development of the placenta, and myometrial contractions.[49] MCs have also been found to produce a variety of inflammatory mediators that may have a role in cervical ripening.[50] However, given the density of MCs in the myometrium, MCs have also been implicated in increased uterine contractility observed in systemic reactions to sensitized individuals. Endometrial biopsies in patients with recurrent pregnancy loss were found to have increased numbers of MCs and proinflammatory mediators compared with controls.[51] These observations may indicate a possible role of MC-mediated uterine contractility leading to preterm labor, particularly in women with mastocytosis. Whether this is true clinically remains unclear based on current literature.[47,49] Collectively, these data support the hypothesis that MCs are involved in the human reproductive cycle, and the changes that occur during pregnancy could affect their activity. However, there are few prospective studies that have sought to evaluate the behavior and function of MC in pregnancy in patients with SM.[47]

Mastocytosis in Pregnancy

ISM, which comprises the largest subgroup of patients with systemic mastocytosis, is often diagnosed at a younger age (median age, 49 years) compared with other hematologic conditions.[43] Therefore, conception and pregnancy may require management during a patient's lifetime. Both pregnancy and labor could induce worsening of mastocytosis symptoms, including flushing, urticaria and pruritis, gastrointestinal symptoms, and anaphylaxis. This has relevant implications for obstetric management and prenatal interdisciplinary care during pregnancy in patients with mastocytosis.[47]

Pregnancy causes significant physical and psychological stressors that can trigger worsening symptoms of mastocytosis in about one-third of patients.[52] In a small series of 12 pregnant patients with mastocytosis, 4 of the 12 women experienced a deterioration in symptoms; 7 patients had no change, and one patient had improvement.[47] Matito and colleagues[53] followed 45 pregnancies in patients with mastocytosis and found in 10 pregnancies (22%) MC-related symptoms worsened; one woman developed new-onset urticaria pigmentosa during the third trimester; and 15 cases (33%) experienced clinical improvement during pregnancy. MC mediator release symptoms were seen intrapartum in 5 cases (11%) with no fatal outcomes.

Management of mastocytosis during pregnancy requires an interdisciplinary team consisting of a high-risk obstetrician, a hematologist, an allergist, and an anesthesiologist.[47] Treatment is directed toward alleviating symptoms while weighing risk of any medications to the fetus.[52] Minimizing MC-mediated symptoms is thought to benefit the patient and reduce risk to the fetus.[49] Use of antimediator drugs, such as antihistamines, corticosteroids, and epinephrine, is considered reasonable during pregnancy. Other options include MC stabilizers, leukotriene antagonists, and omalizumab.[49] Cytoreductive agents with the exception of possibly interferon-α are associated with potential fetal harm and are not recommended.[49]

Management of labor and delivery focuses on prevention and preparation for treatment of anaphylaxis. MC degranulation can occur perioperatively owing to emotion or physical stress, allergen exposures, or drugs that promote the release of histamine if the prior tolerance is unknown.[49] Medications that have been implicated in iatrogenic anaphylaxis include codeine, morphine, certain muscle relaxants, such as mivacurium and atracurium, and some antibiotics (including vancomycin). Alternative agents are typically recommended if a patient's tolerance is unknown to these drugs. Fentanyl, benzodiazepines, and local anesthetics are generally well-tolerated. The neuromuscular blocking agents, succinylcholine and cisatracurium, appear to have the least mastocytosis mediator release effect.[49,54] NSAIDs should also be avoided if prior tolerance is unknown.[49]

In general, the incidence of iatrogenic anaphylaxis in mastocytosis is low. However, some experts still recommend pretreatment of delivery with antihistamines, glucocorticoids, and oral cromolyn sodium.[54] Home births should be avoided, and the patient's medical team should have immediate access to epinephrine, establish intravenous access, and be able to perform resuscitation if shock occurs.[49]

Mastocytosis and Pregnancy Outcomes

The diagnosis of SM does not appear to have any effect on fertility, although few studies exist.[47] All conceptions reported in patients with SM have occurred naturally, aside from one achieved by in vitro fertilization owing to a history of infertility.[53]

Three clinical cases reported onset of preterm labor at 24 to 27 weeks associated with elevated levels of serum and urinary histamine. However, delivery was successfully reached at 36 to 40 weeks in these cases, with 2 cases requiring tocolytics and antihistamines to control premature uterine contractions.[47] In a Polish cohort study, 4 of 23 (17%) pregnancies resulted in preterm birth.[55] However, the larger study by Matito and colleagues[53] did not report detrimental effects of mastocytosis on pregnancy outcomes. No other significant recurrent pregnancy complications that can be specifically attributed to mastocytosis have been reported.[47]

Indolent Systemic Mastocytosis Without Skin Findings Associated with Hymenoptera Venom Anaphylaxis

ISM associated with insect-induced anaphylaxis displays unique clinical, biological, and molecular characteristics as compared with other systemic mastocytosis cases. The prevalence of clonal MC activation diseases, ISM and MMAS, among patients presenting with HVA, ranges from 1% to 7.9%.[56] ISM without skin lesions associated with HVA is characterized by low bone marrow MC burden[45] **(Fig. 1)**. Alvarez-Twose and colleagues,[46] in a 2014 study of one of the largest series of patients with ISM with

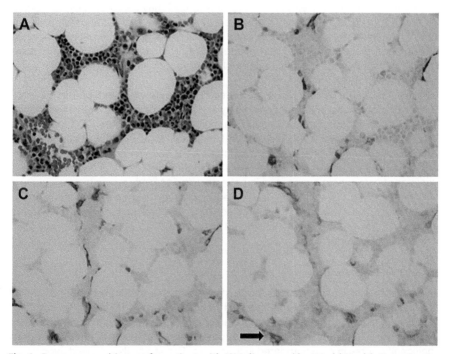

Fig. 1. Bone marrow biopsy of a patient with ISM diagnosed by World Health Organization minor criteria only (lacking MC aggregates). (*A*) Hematoxylin-eosin, original magnification, ×400. (*B*) Tryptase, ×400. MCs are stained brown and have spindle and elongated shapes and are partially degranulated. (*C*) CD117, ×400. (*D*) CD25, x400. (*arrow*) MC shows a characteristic abnormal spindle shape. (*Courtesy of* Charles Ross, MD, Ann Arbor, MI, with permission.)

associated HVA, showed a clear male predominance in this group of patients (78% men vs 22% women). However, no gender predilection was observed in this study among patients with ISM-associated with anaphylaxis triggers other than insects. Zanotti and colleagues[57] similarly found a male predominance (87% men vs 13% women) in 15 patients diagnosed with ISM after at least one episode of HVA associated with hypotension. Interestingly, all patients were diagnosed with ISM based on minor criteria, as none were found to have MC aggregates based on bone marrow biopsy in this study. The median basal serum tryptase was 8.4 ng/mL.

The REMA score is a simple scoring system that considers clinical parameters and serum baseline tryptase that predicts with high sensitivity the diagnosis of ISM.[58] When applying the REMA score to patients with MC activation symptoms related to insect sting, it has been found to have a specificity of 67% and sensitivity of 92%, making it a useful tool for a selection of candidates for further bone marrow evaluation.[46] ISM must be strongly suspected in male patients with cardiovascular vasodilatory-related symptoms or anaphylaxis in the absence of pruritis, urticaria, and angioedema after insect sting independent of serum tryptase levels.[45]

Mastocytosis and Osteoporosis

Up to 50% of patients with mastocytosis are found to have bone involvement in the form of osteopenia or osteoporosis.[59] Prevalence of mastocytosis-related osteoporosis appears to be higher in men (28%) than women (9%).[60] One study showed that the lack of skin involvement in patients with ISM may serve as an independent risk factor for fragility fractures.[61] However, other studies did not find this association.[60,61] A higher prevalence of low bone mineral density (BMD) has been reported in the subgroup of patients with ISM without history of anaphylaxis.[62] Therefore, osteoporosis in the absence of typical skin involvement or triggers for anaphylaxis may be the only sign of ISM.

Fragility fractures, particularly in the vertebral bones, have been found to be associated with decreased bone mineral density and ISM. In one study, the prevalence of at least one vertebral fracture was 20% in men and 14% in women. Often, multiple vertebral fractures were found.[63] In general, male sex, low hip BMD, absence of urticaria pigmentosa, and increased alcohol intake have been found as independent risk factors for future fractures in patients with ISM. Serum tryptase was not found to be a predictor of osteoporosis presence in patients with SM.[62,63]

Taken together, SM should be considered a potential diagnosis in the screening of all premenopausal women and in men presenting with unexplained fragility fractures or low BMD. SM should also be considered in postmenopausal women with suspicion of secondary osteoporosis.[60]

Mastocytosis and Survival

Male patients with ISM have a higher rate of progression and death compared with female patients. A study found overall survival (OS) is worse with ISM compared with CM, and male gender was an independent risk factor for a worse prognosis.[64] When considering all forms of systemic mastocytosis, progression-free survival ($P = .0002$) was significantly worse in men compared with women. This study also showed overall survival ($P<.001$) was significantly inferior in men. A median overall survival difference of 11 years (17.4 vs 28.4 years) was seen in female patients. Worse outcomes in male patients with SM are thought to be due to increased cytogenetic and molecular abnormalities. These may be related to sex hormones or lifestyle factors, such as smoking, which may increase acquisition of mutations in neoplastic progenitor cells in SM.[65]

CLINICS CARE POINTS

- Incidence of anaphylaxis is increased in female patients compared with male patients in pubertal years, but this disparity narrows after later middle age.
- Sex hormones are implicated in rare causes of anaphylaxis, such as catamenial, progestogen, and lactation anaphylaxis.
- Estrogen worsens passive anaphylaxis in mouse models by increasing tissue expression of endothelial nitric oxide synthase, which increases vascular permeability.
- Indolent systemic mastocytosis does not appear to affect fertility or pregnancy outcomes but should be managed by a multidisciplinary team with a focus on symptom prevention while minimizing risk to the fetus.
- Incidence of systemic mastocytosis is increased in women; however, disease-free progression and overall survival are significantly worse in men owing to increased cytogenetic and molecular abnormalities.

DISCLOSURE

S.S. Ellingwood: No disclosures. A. Kovalszki: Blueprint Medicines Co-Investigator on PIONEER, PROSPECTOR, and HARBOR trials, Cogent Biosciences Co-Investigator on SUMMIT trial.

REFERENCES

1. González-Pérez A, Aponte Z, Vidaurre CF, et al. Anaphylaxis epidemiology in patients with and patients without asthma: A United Kingdom database review. J Allergy Clin Immunol 2010;125(5):1098–104.e1.
2. Ross MP, Ferguson M, Street D, et al. Analysis of food-allergic and anaphylactic events in the National Electronic Injury Surveillance System. J Allergy Clin Immunol 2008;121(1):166–71.
3. Webb LM, Lieberman P. Anaphylaxis: a review of 601 cases. Ann Allergy Asthma Immunol 2006;97(1):39–43.
4. Voltolini S, Cofini V, Murzilli F, et al. Hypersensitivity reactions to iodinate contrast media in Italy: a retrospective study. Characteristics of patients and risk factors. Eur Ann Allergy Clin Immunol 2022;54(02):60.
5. Kvedariene V, Martins P, Rouanet L, et al. Diagnosis of iodinated contrast media hypersensitivity: results of a 6-year period. Clin Exp Allergy J Br Soc Allergy Clin Immunol 2006;36(8):1072–7.
6. Chen W, Mempel M, Schober W, et al. Gender difference, sex hormones, and immediate type hypersensitivity reactions. Allergy 2008;63(11):1418–27.
7. International Collaborative Study of Severe Anaphylaxis. Risk of anaphylaxis in a hospital population in relation to the use of various drugs: an international study. Pharmacoepidemiol Drug Saf 2003;12(3):195–202.
8. Imai K, Tanaka F, Kawano S, et al. Incidence and Risk Factors of Immediate Hypersensitivity Reactions and Immunization Stress-Related Responses With COVID-19 mRNA Vaccine. J Allergy Clin Immunol Pract 2022;10(10):2667–76.e10.
9. Alhumaid S, Al Mutair A, Al Alawi Z, et al. Anaphylactic and nonanaphylactic reactions to SARS-CoV-2 vaccines: a systematic review and meta-analysis. Allergy Asthma Clin Immunol 2021;17(1):109.
10. Fenny N, Grammer LC. Idiopathic anaphylaxis. Immunol Allergy Clin North Am 2015;35(2):349–62.

11. Hox V, Desai A, Bandara G, et al. Estrogen increases the severity of anaphylaxis in female mice through enhanced endothelial nitric oxide synthase expression and nitric oxide production. J Allergy Clin Immunol 2015;135(3):729–36.e5.

12. Lin K, Rasheed A, Lin S, et al. Catamenial anaphylaxis: a woman under monthly progesterone curse. Case Rep 2018;2018. https://doi.org/10.1136/bcr-2017-222047. bcr.

13. Buchheit KM, Bernstein JA. Progestogen Hypersensitivity: Heterogeneous Manifestations with a Common Trigger. J Allergy Clin Immunol Pract 2017;5(3):566–74.

14. Carra S, Schatz M, Mertes PM, et al. Anaphylaxis and Pregnancy: A Systematic Review and Call for Public Health Actions. J Allergy Clin Immunol Pract 2021;9(12):4270–8.

15. Zaitsu M, Narita SI, Lambert KC, et al. Estradiol activates mast cells via a nongenomic estrogen receptor-alpha and calcium influx. Mol Immunol 2007;44(8):1977–85.

16. Salvati L, Vitiello G, Parronchi P. Gender differences in anaphylaxis. Curr Opin Allergy Clin Immunol 2019;19(5):417–24.

17. Mackey E, Ayyadurai S, Pohl CS, et al. Sexual dimorphism in the mast cell transcriptome and the pathophysiological responses to immunological and psychological stress. Biol Sex Differ 2016;7:60.

18. Vasiadi M, Kempuraj D, Boucher W, et al. Progesterone inhibits mast cell secretion. Int J Immunopathol Pharmacol 2006;19(4). https://doi.org/10.1177/039463200601900408.

19. Zierau O, Zenclussen AC, Jensen F. Role of female sex hormones, estradiol and progesterone, in mast cell behavior. Front Immunol 2012;3:169.

20. Chen W, Beck I, Schober W, et al. Human mast cells express androgen receptors but treatment with testosterone exerts no influence on IgE-independent mast cell degranulation elicited by neuromuscular blocking agents. Exp Dermatol 2010;19(3):302–4.

21. Guhl S, Artuc M, Zuberbier T, et al. Testosterone exerts selective anti-inflammatory effects on human skin mast cells in a cell subset dependent manner. Exp Dermatol 2012;21(11):878–80.

22. Jensen-Jarolim E, Untersmayr E. Gender-medicine aspects in allergology. Allergy 2008;63(5):610–5.

23. Kulthanan K, Ungprasert P, Jirapongsananuruk O, et al. Food-Dependent Exercise-Induced Wheals, Angioedema, and Anaphylaxis: A Systematic Review. J Allergy Clin Immunol Pract 2022;10(9):2280–96.

24. Pali-Schöll I, Jensen-Jarolim E. Gender aspects in food allergy. Curr Opin Allergy Clin Immunol 2019;19(3):249–55.

25. McNeil MM, DeStefano F. Vaccine-associated hypersensitivity. J Allergy Clin Immunol 2018;141(2):463–72.

26. Yu RJ, Krantz MS, Phillips EJ, et al. Emerging Causes of Drug-Induced Anaphylaxis: A Review of Anaphylaxis-Associated Reports in the FDA Adverse Event Reporting System (FAERS). J Allergy Clin Immunol Pract 2021;9(2):819–29.e2.

27. Sloane D, Govindarajulu U, Harrow-Mortelliti J, et al. Safety, Costs, and Efficacy of Rapid Drug Desensitizations to Chemotherapy and Monoclonal Antibodies. J Allergy Clin Immunol Pract 2016;4(3):497–504.

28. Castells M. Drug Hypersensitivity and Anaphylaxis in Cancer and Chronic Inflammatory Diseases: The Role of Desensitizations. Front Immunol 2017;8:1472.

29. Galvão VR, Phillips E, Giavina-Bianchi P, et al. Carboplatin-allergic patients undergoing desensitization: prevalence and impact of the BRCA 1/2 mutation. J Allergy Clin Immunol Pract 2017;5(3):816–8.

30. Stoevesandt J, Sturm GJ, Bonadonna P, et al. Risk factors and indicators of severe systemic insect sting reactions. Allergy 2020;75(3):535–45.
31. Fisher DA. Drug-induced progesterone dermatitis. J Am Acad Dermatol 1996; 34(5, Part 1):863–4.
32. Baptist AP, Baldwin JL. Autoimmune progesterone dermatitis in a patient with endometriosis: case report and review of the literature. Clin Mol Allergy CMA 2004;2(1):10.
33. Bauer CS, Kampitak T, Messieh ML, et al. Heterogeneity in presentation and treatment of catamenial anaphylaxis. Ann Allergy Asthma Immunol 2013;111(2): 107–11.
34. Burstein M, Rubinow A, Shalit M. Cyclic anaphylaxis associated with menstruation. Ann Allergy 1991;66(1):36–8.
35. Durgakeri P, Jones B. A rare case of lactation anaphylaxis. Australas Med J 2015; 8(3):103–5.
36. McKinney KK, Scranton SE. A case report of breastfeeding anaphylaxis: successful prophylaxis with oral antihistamines. Allergy 2011;66(3):435–6.
37. Shank JJ, Olney SC, Lin FL, et al. Recurrent postpartum anaphylaxis with breastfeeding. Obstet Gynecol 2009;114(2 Pt 2):415–6.
38. Mullins RJ, Russell A, McGrath GJ, et al. Breastfeeding anaphylaxis. Lancet 1991;338(8777):1279–80.
39. Greenberger PA, Lieberman P. Idiopathic anaphylaxis. J Allergy Clin Immunol Pract 2014;2(3):243–50 [quiz: 251].
40. Mikhail I, Stukus DR, Prince BT. Fatal Anaphylaxis: Epidemiology and Risk Factors. Curr Allergy Asthma Rep 2021;21(4):28.
41. Turner PJ, Jerschow E, Umasunthar T, et al. Fatal Anaphylaxis: Mortality Rate and Risk Factors. J Allergy Clin Immunol Pract 2017;5(5):1169–78.
42. Jerschow E, Lin RY, Scaperotti MM, et al. Fatal anaphylaxis in the United States, 1999-2010: temporal patterns and demographic associations. J Allergy Clin Immunol 2014;134(6):1318–28.e7.
43. Pardanani A. Systemic mastocytosis in adults: 2021 Update on diagnosis, risk stratification and management. Am J Hematol 2021;96(4):508–25.
44. Cohen SS, Skovbo S, Vestergaard H, et al. Epidemiology of systemic mastocytosis in Denmark. Br J Haematol 2014;166(4):521–8.
45. Alvarez-Twose I, Matito A. Mastocytosis presenting as insect anaphylaxis: gender differences and natural history. Curr Opin Allergy Clin Immunol 2019;19(5): 468–74.
46. Alvarez-Twose I, Zanotti R, González-de-Olano D, et al. Nonaggressive systemic mastocytosis (SM) without skin lesions associated with insect-induced anaphylaxis shows unique features versus other indolent SM. J Allergy Clin Immunol 2014;133(2):520–8.
47. Ferrari J, Benvenuti P, Bono E, et al. Fertility and Pregnancy Management in a Rare Disease. Front Oncol 2022;12:874178.
48. Jensen F, Woudwyk M, Teles A, et al. Estradiol and progesterone regulate the migration of mast cells from the periphery to the uterus and induce their maturation and degranulation. PLoS One 2010;5(12):e14409.
49. Arora N, Akin C, Kovalszki A. Mastocytosis in Pregnancy. Immunol Allergy Clin North Am 2023;43(1):159–68.
50. Norström A, Vukas Radulovic N, Bullarbo M, et al. Mast cell involvement in human cervical ripening. Eur J Obstet Gynecol Reprod Biol 2019;238:157–63.

51. Derbala Y, Elazzamy H, Bilal M, et al. Mast cell–induced immunopathology in recurrent pregnancy losses. Am J Reprod Immunol 2019;82(1). https://doi.org/10.1111/aji.13128.
52. Lei D, Akin C, Kovalszki A. Management of Mastocytosis in Pregnancy: A Review. J Allergy Clin Immunol Pract 2017;5(5):1217–23.
53. Matito A, Álvarez-Twose I, Morgado JM, et al. Clinical impact of pregnancy in mastocytosis: a study of the Spanish Network on Mastocytosis (REMA) in 45 cases. Int Arch Allergy Immunol 2011;156(1):104–11.
54. Hermans MAW, Arends NJT, Gerth van Wijk R, et al. Management around invasive procedures in mastocytosis: An update. Ann Allergy Asthma Immunol 2017;119(4):304–9.
55. Ciach K, Niedoszytko M, Abacjew-Chmylko A, et al. Pregnancy and Delivery in Patients with Mastocytosis Treated at the Polish Center of the European Competence Network on Mastocytosis (ECNM). PLoS One 2016;11(1):e0146924.
56. Bonadonna P, Scaffidi L. Hymenoptera Anaphylaxis as a Clonal Mast Cell Disorder. Immunol Allergy Clin North Am 2018;38(3):455–68.
57. Zanotti R, Lombardo C, Passalacqua G, et al. Clonal mast cell disorders in patients with severe Hymenoptera venom allergy and normal serum tryptase levels. J Allergy Clin Immunol 2015;136(1):135–9.
58. Alvarez-Twose I, González-de-Olano D, Sánchez-Muñoz L, et al. Validation of the REMA score for predicting mast cell clonality and systemic mastocytosis in patients with systemic mast cell activation symptoms. Int Arch Allergy Immunol 2012;157(3):275–80.
59. Barete S, Assous N, de Gennes C, et al. Systemic mastocytosis and bone involvement in a cohort of 75 patients. Ann Rheum Dis 2010;69(10):1838–41.
60. Rossini M, Zanotti R, Orsolini G, et al. Prevalence, pathogenesis, and treatment options for mastocytosis-related osteoporosis. Osteoporos Int 2016;27(8):2411–21.
61. van der Veer E, van der Goot W, de Monchy JGR, et al. High prevalence of fractures and osteoporosis in patients with indolent systemic mastocytosis. Allergy 2012;67(3):431–8.
62. Rossini M, Zanotti R, Bonadonna P, et al. Bone mineral density, bone turnover markers and fractures in patients with indolent systemic mastocytosis. Bone 2011;49(4):880–5.
63. Rossini M, Zanotti R, Viapiana O, et al. Bone involvement and osteoporosis in mastocytosis. Immunol Allergy Clin North Am 2014;34(2):383–96.
64. Trizuljak J, Sperr WR, Nekvindová L, et al. Clinical features and survival of patients with indolent systemic mastocytosis defined by the updated WHO classification. Allergy Eur J Allergy Clin Immunol 2020;75(8):1923–34.
65. Kluin-Nelemans HC, Jawhar M, Reiter A, et al. Cytogenetic and molecular aberrations and worse outcome for male patients in systemic mastocytosis. Theranostics 2021;11(1):292–303.
66. Muñoz-Cruz S, Mendoza-Rodríguez Y, Nava-Castro KE, et al. Gender-related effects of sex steroids on histamine release and FcεRI expression in rat peritoneal mast cells. J Immunol Res 2015;2015. https://doi.org/10.1155/2015/351829.

Update on Mast Cell Proteases as Drug Targets

George H. Caughey, MD*

KEYWORDS

- Tryptase • Chymase • Cathepsin G • Dipeptidyl peptidase-I • Cathepsin C
- Carboxypeptidase A3

KEY POINTS

- Mast cells secrete proteases with hypothesized roles in host defense and disease.
- Preclinical models suggest that inactivation of one or more mast cell proteases lessen pathologies associated with allergy, inflammation, and recovery from injury.
- Pharmacologic inhibitors of human β-tryptases, chymase, cathepsin G, and dipeptidyl peptidase-I have been developed and tested.
- Human studies suggest that β-tryptases, chymase, or dipeptidyl peptidase-I can be safely inactivated, implying dispensable short-term roles in homeostasis and host defense.
- Inhibition of dipeptidyl peptidase-I, which also is produced by other granulated leukocytes, improved bronchiectasis in a human trial.

INTRODUCTION

Human mast cells make, store, and secrete proteases regarded as targets for drug development, as previously reviewed.[1–3] Some of these, such as tryptases, chymase, and carboxypeptidase A3, are exclusive to mast cells or nearly so. Others, such as cathepsin G and dipeptidyl peptidase-I (cathepsin C), also appear in other cell types, such as neutrophils. Mast cell secretory granules are well endowed with β-tryptases, which are abundant proteins in nearly all mature, granulated human mast cells. Expression of mast cell chymase, cathepsin G, and carboxypeptidase A3 protein, however, is restricted to a subset of cells in several tissue sites, especially dermis, and may increase in other organs subject to scarring, as in fibrotic lung, heart, and kidney.

Over the past half-century, many studies defined and explored the nature, variation, expression, secretion, enzymology, evolution, and biological functions of mammalian mast cell proteases. The results engendered a range of hypotheses regarding contributions to tissue homeostasis, immunity, inflammation, and pathobiology. Yet, as for mast cells in general, the importance of proteases relative to other components of host

University of California at San Francisco
* Department of Medicine, 533 Parnassus Avenue, San Francisco, CA 94143, USA.
E-mail address: george.caughey@ucsf.edu

Immunol Allergy Clin N Am 43 (2023) 777–787
https://doi.org/10.1016/j.iac.2023.04.006
0889-8561/23/© 2023 Elsevier Inc. All rights reserved.
immunology.theclinics.com

defense remain something of a cipher. In part because extracellular proteases can be destructive, many investigators predicted that proteases released from mast cells are pro-inflammatory and are logical targets for therapeutic inhibition to limit inflammation. Other investigators, especially those exploring mast cell biology in mice, posited important and perhaps essential roles in innate immunity, host defense against parasites, tissue repair following injury, and detoxification of venoms and endogenous peptides, pointing to potential downsides of inactivation. Selected proteases became the focus of pharmaceutical development of inhibitors for use in humans. After years of preclinical testing—and stops and starts—several inhibitors reached the point of testing in humans. Some of these are reviewed briefly here. Other studies are ongoing. We can expect to learn more concerning benefits and drawbacks of inhibition as well as about roles of specific proteases and mast cells overall as results are available.

TRYPTASES: ABUNDANCE, MULTIPLICITY, AND GENETIC VARIATION

Tryptases receive the lion's share of attention among mast cell proteases. Partly, this is because they are abundant in almost all mature human mast cells, exploited by pathologists in the histochemical detection of mast cells, and used as biomarkers of mast cell biomass and activation disorders, including mastocytosis and anaphylaxis. However, tryptases also are more diverse, complex, and genetically variable than the other proteases, which frustrates targeting and testing of inhibitors in conditions such as asthma, allergic rhinitis, urticaria, and inflammatory bowel disease.[1,2,4] Tryptases have been considered not solely as targets for inactivation, but as therapeutic agents in their own right because of a capacity to detoxify snake venoms[5] (**Fig. 1**).

Human tryptases are products of four clustered genes: TPSAB1, TPSB2, TPSD1, and TPSG1. The focus is on inhibiting β-tryptases, which are products of genes at two sites: TPSAB1 and TPSB2.[6] However, genetic variation in this regard is substantial. Active β-tryptases are soluble, heparin-bound, toroidal tetramers[7] stored preactivated in secretory granules and exocytosed in response to stimuli that release histamine from the same granules.[8] Individuals in most human populations inherit as few as two or as many as four genes encoding active β-tryptases,[9] and mast cells from individuals inheriting more active genes appear to contain more active tryptase.[10] Some β-tryptases are inactive, such as a frame-shifted variant that is common in populations of European origin.[9] To further muddy the landscape of tryptase inheritance, genes encoding α-tryptases usually compete with β genes as alleles at TPSAB1, which matters because α-tryptases by themselves are catalytically minimally active or inactive.[11] However, α-tryptases alter β-subunit activity if incorporated into a tetramer, enhancing ability to activate targets such as mechanosensory and protease-activated receptors implicated in vibratory urticaria, pain, and itch.[12] In this regard, the finding that α-tryptase genes are absent in up to a half of chromosomes in populations of European and African origin[9,13] may be clinically significant. Individuals without α-genes usually inherit active β-genes instead[9] (**Fig. 2**).

Even though some chromosomes lack α-genes, others host one or more extra copies of a TPSAB1 gene encoding α-tryptase. Typically, this results in elevated baseline levels of circulating immunoreactive tryptase, that is, hereditary α-tryptasemia.[14] Although not as common as hereditary absence of α-tryptase, hereditary α-tryptasemia affects about one in 20 individuals in White populations, and the frequency is higher in individuals with mastocytosis and serious sensitivity to hymenoptera stings, as previously reviewed.[15] Although much has been written in recent years about α-tryptase inheritance and influence on baseline levels of immunoreactive tryptase, these proteins have not been targeted for development of active-site inhibitors

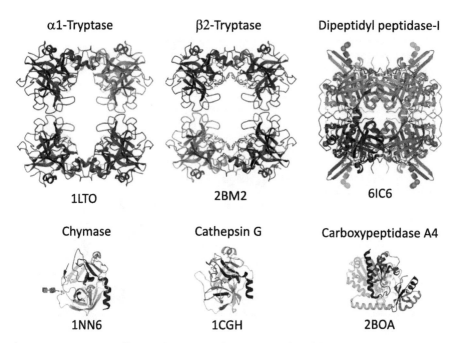

α1-Tryptase   β2-Tryptase   Dipeptidyl peptidase-I

1LTO   2BM2   6IC6

Chymase   Cathepsin G   Carboxypeptidase A4

1NN6   1CGH   2BOA

Fig. 1. Human mast cell granule-associated proteases. The ribbon structures are crystal-based models of the natively blocked α_1-tryptase tetramer (Protein Database identifier 1LTO), the β_2-tryptase tetramer with inward-facing active sites bridged and blocked by bifunctional inhibitors (2BM2); the dipeptidyl peptidase-I tetramer with outward-facing active sites (6IC6); the prochymase monomer with attached N-linked sugars (1NN6), the cathepsin G monomer with active site blocked by an irreversible peptidic inhibitor (1CGH), and carboxypeptidase A4 (2BOA) as a stand-in for carboxypeptidase A3, for which no crystal-based structure is available.

because, as noted, they are already catalytically impaired. This is also true of TPSD1-generated δ-tryptases, which are severely truncated,[6] although they are full-length and active in some nonhuman primates serving as preclinical models of asthma and other conditions.[16] Products of the TPSG1 gene, the transmembrane, or γ-tryptases are membrane-anchored, insoluble on release, and apparently expressed by a minority of human mast cells. Consequently, they receive less attention than soluble α/β-tryptases,[17] although they have pro-inflammatory potential if expressed in soluble form and injected into mouse airway.[18] Intriguingly, mice lacking the TPSG1 gene exhibit increased baseline airway reactivity to methacholine but reduced severity of cigarette smoke-induced chronic obstructive lung disease,[19] which can be interpreted as either beneficial or deleterious or both. The importance of γ-tryptases to animals in general is unclear because the gene is absent in many mammals.[17]

PHARMACOLOGIC INACTIVATION OF β-TRYPTASES

Inhibitors of human β-tryptases were explored initially decades ago. An early test was a small, randomized, double-blinded crossover study of subjects with mild atopic asthma.[20] The study drug (Arris Pharmaceutical Company [APC] 366) was a slow-acting small molecule delivered to airways by aerosol inhalation and was not specific for tryptases. Although the clinical benefit was modest, the finding that APC 366

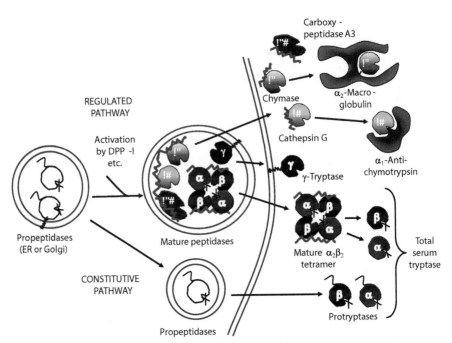

Fig. 2. Biogenesis and fate of secreted human mast cell proteases. In presecretory organelles, proteases are activated from zymogens by dipeptidyl peptidase-I (DPP-I) and other pro-peptide processing enzymes. In a regulated secretory pathway, mature chymase (Ch), cathepsin G (CG), carboxypeptidase A3 (CPA), and tryptases are packaged in granules with heparin and other proteoglycans (blue *lines*). γ-Tryptase is attached to granule membrane via a C-terminal transmembrane peptide. Following degranulation, it is anchored to the extracellular surface. After propeptide removal, β-tryptases form tetramers of two or more types of β or α/βcombinations. Proteases not activated from pro-forms are released by a constitutive pathway. Following exocytosis, cathepsin G and chymase are inhibited by α_1-antichymotrypsin and α_2-macroglobulin, respectively, with chymase retaining ability to cleave small peptides after capture. Secreted tryptase tetramers resist anti-proteases but lose activity by dissociating into inactive monomers. All secreted α- and β-tryptases, including pro-forms, contribute to levels of immunoreactive tryptase measured in clinically employed assays.

reduced late asthmatic responses to inhaled allergen was consistent with a potential role for tryptases or related airway proteases in asthma. Another nonspecific inhibitor of β-tryptases tested in humans with allergic airway disease was Robert Wood Johnson (RWJ)-58643, a potent, reversible, competitive inhibitor of β-tryptases and pancreatic trypsin. This inhibitor was tested by topical nasal administration in a randomized, double-blind, single-center four-way crossover study of 16 subjects with allergic rhinitis challenged out of season with grass pollen.[21] The study drug reduced symptoms and eosinophilia at low doses after nasal allergen challenge compared with placebo, but higher doses of RWJ-58643 increased eosinophilia. As with the APC 366 study, this study was interpreted as therapeutically somewhat promising and consistent with a role for mast cell β-tryptases in allergic airway inflammation, but inconclusive without high-level specificity of the drugs for the mast cell enzymes.

Numerous alternative pharmacologic approaches to β-tryptase inhibition have been explored, including developing orally bioavailable anti-tryptases, addressing the challenge of inactivating tryptases inside of granules prior to release, and achieving high-level specificity by bridging active sites across the "donut-hole" of the tetramer using self-assembling heterodimeric inhibitors.[22] Some candidate inhibitors have been tested in preclinical models of asthma and other conditions, as previously reviewed.[1,2,4] The most recent approach to reach the point of testing in humans used antibodies as "molecular pliers" to dissociate active subunits of secreted β-tryptase tetramer into inactive monomers.[10] This strategy of destabilizing tetramers was first explored over two decades ago in a less tryptase-selective manner using antagonists of heparin, which is attached to and stabilizes the tetramer on release from mast cells.[23,24] A Phase I study of tetramer-dissociating antibody MTPS9579A demonstrated safety and biochemical efficacy, namely suppression of upper airway β-tryptase activity in subjects injected with antibody.[25] A Phase IIa multicenter, randomized, placebo-controlled, double-blind study of this antibody in 135 subjects with moderate to severe uncontrolled asthma further exploring efficacy, safety, and pharmacokinetics is registered with Clinicaltrials.gov (Identifier NCT04092582). Results of this trial, listed complete as of May 2022, are not yet published as this is written.

Another early target of anti-tryptases was inflammatory bowel disease, which first was tested in humans using the selective small-molecule inhibitor APC 2059 in a multicenter, open-label study without a placebo arm in 56 subjects with ulcerative colitis.[26] The drug was subcutaneously injected twice daily for 4 weeks. Nearly half of subjects improved in parameters of disease activity, suggesting a potential therapeutic benefit. However, further development of APC 2059 for this indication was discontinued in the context of refocusing resources on development of anti-tryptases with oral bioavailability. Later case reports recording improvement in ulcerative colitis from enemas containing nafamostat speculatively attributed the response to tryptase inhibition.[27] Nafamostat is a potent, slowly reversible suicide inhibitor of β-tryptases,[28] but also inactivates a range of other tryptic serine proteases,[29] making it hazardous to assign full credit to tryptase inhibition for observed therapeutic effects.

CHYMASE

In contrast to mice and rat genomes, which harbor large clusters of chymase-related protease genes, human genomes contain one chymase-expressing gene, CMA1, as previously summarized.[30] The multiplicity of rodent chymase-like genes and their varying substrate specificities have complicated preclinical modeling of human chymase function and inhibition in mice and rats. Notable activities of human chymase, a serine-class protease with preferences similar but not identical to those of chymotrypsin, include angiotensin converting enzyme-independent generation of angiotensin II and activation of transforming growth factor (TGF)β1 and matrix metalloproteinases, consistent with potential roles in blood pressure control, wound healing, remodeling, and fibrosis. The first selective chymase inhibitor to reach human trials was fulacimstat. Phase I studies of oral drug showed minimal adverse effects in healthy humans and subjects with ischemic heart disease and no blood pressure drop.[31,32] On this basis, fulacimstat advanced to 6-month, multinational, double-blind, randomized, placebo-controlled trials. However, the drug did not improve cardiac performance in humans with left ventricular dysfunction following myocardial infarction[33], nor did it prevent progression of albuminuria in subjects with type 2 diabetes-associated kidney disease.[34] These studies, while suggesting that systemic inhibition of chymase is safe, have yet to identify a therapeutic benefit. Thus, human mast cell chymase remains a target in search of a disease.

CATHEPSIN G AND DIPEPTIDYL PEPTIDASE-I

Human cathepsin G, a serine-class protease related to chymase and expressed by chymase gene CMA1's near-neighbor cathepsin G (CTSG), differs from human chymase in key attributes.[35] In contrast to mouse cathepsin G, which has an activity profile highly akin to that of chymotryptic chymases, the human enzyme's suite of active-site mutations acquired during primate evolution[36] resulted in a potentially more destructive profile, including tryptic, elastolytic, and met-ase activity. Cathepsin G's fate after release from cells also differs from that of chymase, in which it is inactivated in blood irreversibly by α_1-antichymotrypsin, whereas human chymase is captured within the α_2-macroglobulin cage, within which it retains ability to cleave small substrates, including angiotensin I.[37] Unlike chymase, cathepsin G is expressed by neutrophils as well as by mast cells. However, in the subset of human mast cells that express cathepsin G, the enzyme is abundant with levels approximating those of chymase.[38] The proposed roles for human cathepsin G include tissue damage, inflammation, formation of neutrophil extracellular traps, and antibacterial defenses.[3]

Dual inhibitors of cathepsin G and mast cell chymase have been developed and tested in preclinical models of human disease, including lung inflammation.[39] To this reviewer's knowledge, no selective, direct inhibitors of cathepsin G have reached advanced stages of preclinical testing or clinical trials. However, drugs that block cathepsin G and related proenzyme activation from zymogens have been tested. One of these, GSK2793660, an oral irreversible inhibitor of dipeptidyl peptidase-I (cathepsin C), achieved ∼90% inhibition of the target enzyme in whole blood and a lesser decrease in activity of circulating cathepsin G. These results were obtained in a Phase I randomized placebo-controlled crossover study of healthy male subjects.[40] However, 7 of 10 subjects receiving repeat doses of the inhibitor manifested epithelial desquamation of palmar and plantar surfaces of hands and feet, which was suspected to be related to inhibition of dipeptidyl peptidase-I because of high frequency in subjects receiving the drug and because humans with genetic deficiencies in dipeptidyl peptidase-I develop palmoplantar skin lesions early in life.[41]

Another dipeptidyl peptidase-I inhibitor, brensocatib (which, in contrast to GSK2793660, is reversible) also was tested as an anti-inflammatory agent preventing activation and expression of neutrophil cathepsin G, elastase, and proteinase-3, as previously reviewed.[3] In WILLOW, a 6-month multinational double-blind, randomized placebo-controlled trial in humans with non-cystic fibrosis bronchiectasis, brensocatib was safe and well tolerated, and achieved the primary endpoint of prolonging time to first exacerbation.[42] A phase 3 trial is registered with clinicaltrials.gov in non-cystic bronchiectasis (trial identifier NCT04594369), along with a phase IIa trial (trial identifier NCT05090904) in bronchiectasis associated with cystic fibrosis. Although cathepsin G expressed by mast cells was not specifically targeted in these studies, it is likely that the mast cell enzyme is affected. Brensocatib likely also blocks activation of chymase. Although this possibility has not been explored in human mast cells, chymase activity in mast cells is nearly undetectable in mice genetically deficient in dipeptidyl peptidase-I.[43] Mast cell tryptase (mouse mast celll protease [mMCP]-6) activity in these mice is not affected as profoundly as chymase. In vitro studies in human mast cells suggest that this also is the case for human β-tryptases, as alternative cysteine-class cathepsins such as B and L can remove the tryptase propeptide,[44] perhaps processively. β-Tryptase propeptides, which must be cleaved from monomeric zymogens before formation of active tetramers, are substantially longer than the two-residue propeptides of cathepsin G and chymase,[45] which are removed by dipeptidyl peptidase-I in a single step.

CARBOXYPEPTIDASE A3

The mast cell-selective secretory granule protein carboxypeptidase A3, encoded by gene CPA3, is a zinc-dependent exopeptidase belonging to a mechanistic and evolutionary class of hydrolases distinct from those of the serine- and cysteine-class proteases already discussed.[46–48] It removes a C-terminal amino acid from target proteins and peptides, preferring aromatic or hydrophobic residues.[49] Perhaps not coincidentally, these are the residues most often generated at carboxyl termini by the action of chymase or cathepsin G.[50,51] In humans, carboxypeptidase A3 protein expression seems to be limited to the subset of mast cells expressing chymase and cathepsin G[52] with which it segregates in granules.[53] Carboxypeptidase A3 and chymases can exhibit codependence for packaging and degradation of potential targets, such as lipoproteins, toxic venoms, and neuropeptides.[1,50,54,55] Indeed, deletion of the CPA3 gene in mice leads to loss not only of CPA3 in mast cell granules, but also of selected chymase-like enzymes.[54]

Certain endotypes of asthma and allergic rhinitis feature a subset of airway mast cells expressing CPA3 messenger RNA (mRNA) transcripts while apparently lacking the peptidase in granules.[56–58] CPA3 transcripts also are one of six biomarkers forming a "signature" predicting treatment responses in stable asthma and future exacerbations in poorly controlled asthma.[59] Although carboxypeptidase A3 may play roles in detoxification based in vitro studies with human enzyme and in vivo assessment in rodents,[1] its contributions and importance in human tissue homeostasis and allergic inflammation remain to be determined. Relative to tryptases and chymases, progress in discerning the functions of carboxypeptidase A3 is hampered by lack of detailed insights into protein structure and a dearth of highly selective inhibitors with which to explore its potential as a drug target. Enthusiasm for development of inhibitors for clinical use in humans also is dampened by evidence from mice that carboxypeptidase A3 activity can be protective with the implication that inhibition could be deleterious if the enzyme provides similar services for humans. An intriguing finding in mice engineered to express Cre recombinase under control of the CPA3 promoter was a profound decrease in mast cells and a milder decrease in basophils.[60] In addition to creating a useful mast cell deficiency model (Cre-Master mice), this result suggested a potential genetic strategy to achieve mast cell ablation in humans. The unexpected phenotype was attributed to Trp53-dependent genotoxicity rather than to a deficit of carboxypeptidase A3 itself. At this point, to this reviewer's knowledge, no selective inhibitors of mast cell carboxypeptidase A3 have been developed or reached the stage of preclinical or clinical testing.

SUMMARY

Several inhibitors of mast cell secretory granule-associated endo- and exo-peptidases have achieved drug-like status, met benchmarks of preclinical validation, and proceeded to clinical testing in humans. As this is written, the most advanced targets for inhibition are β-tryptases, chymase, and dipeptidyl peptidase-I. Further studies are needed to determine whether targeting one or more of these proteolytic enzymes of mast cell origin offers clinical advantages over other therapies targeting mast cells and their secreted products.

CLINICS CARE POINTS

- Early-phase clinical studies in humans suggest that inhibition of β-tryptases is safe and may be beneficial in asthma, allergic rhinitis, and inflammatory bowel disease.

- Inhibitors of mast cell chymase studied in Phase II clinical trials are safe but show no benefit in post-myocardial infarction ventricular remodeling or diabetic kidney dysfunction.

- Human studies in bronchiectasis suggest that inhibition of dipeptidyl peptidase-I reduces exacerbations, although it is unclear whether enzyme originating from mast cells contributes to this effect.

DISCLOSURES

Consulted for Insmed.

REFERENCES

1. Galli SJ, Tsai M, Marichal T, et al. Approaches for analyzing the roles of mast cells and their proteases in vivo. Adv Immunol 2015;126:46–127.
2. Caughey GH. Mast cell proteases as pharmacological targets. Eur J Pharmacol 2016;778:44–55.
3. Korkmaz B, Caughey GH, Chapple I, et al. Therapeutic targeting of cathepsin C: from pathophysiology to treatment. Pharmacol Ther 2018;190:202–36.
4. Cairns JA. Inhibitors of mast cell tryptase beta as therapeutics for the treatment of asthma and inflammatory disorders. Pulm Pharmacol Ther 2005;18(1):55–66.
5. Anderson E, Stavenhagen K, Kolarich D, et al. Human mast cell tryptase is a potential treatment for snakebite envenoming across multiple snake species. Front Immunol 2018;9:1532.
6. Pallaoro M, Fejzo MS, Shayesteh L, et al. Characterization of genes encoding known and novel human tryptases on chromosome 16p13.3. J Biol Chem 1999;274(6):3355–62.
7. Pereira PJ, Bergner A, Macedo-Ribeiro S, et al. Human beta-tryptase is a ring-like tetramer with active sites facing a central pore. Nature 1998;392(6673):306–11.
8. Schwartz LB, Atkins PC, Bradford TR, et al. Release of tryptase together with histamine during the immediate cutaneous response to allergen. J Allergy Clin Immunol 1987;80(6):850–5.
9. Trivedi NN, Tamraz B, Chu C, et al. Human subjects are protected from mast cell tryptase deficiency despite frequent inheritance of loss-of-function mutations. J Allergy Clin Immunol 2009;124(5):1099–105.
10. Maun HR, Jackman JK, Choy DF, et al. An allosteric anti-tryptase antibody for the treatment of mast cell-mediated severe asthma. Cell 2019;179(2):417–31.
11. Marquardt U, Zettl F, Huber R, et al. The crystal structure of human alpha1-tryptase reveals a blocked substrate-binding region. J Mol Biol 2002;321(3):491–502.
12. Le QT, Lyons JJ, Naranjo AN, et al. Impact of naturally forming human α/β-tryptase heterotetramers in the pathogenesis of hereditary α-tryptasemia. J Exp Med 2019;216(10):2348–61.
13. Soto D, Malmsten C, Blount JL, et al. Genetic deficiency of human mast cell alpha-tryptase. Clin Exp Allergy 2002;32(7):1000–6.
14. Lyons JL, Yu X, Hughes JD, et al. Elevated basal serum tryptase identifies a multisystem disorder associated with increased TPSAB1 copy number. Nat Genet 2016;48(12):1564–9.
15. Glover SC, Carter MC, Korosec P, et al. Clinical relevance of inherited genetic differences in human tryptases: Hereditary alpha-tryptasemia and beyond. Ann Allergy Asthma Immunol 2021;127(6):638–47.

16. Trivedi NN, Raymond WW, Caughey GH. Chimerism, point mutation and truncation dramatically transformed mast cell delta-tryptases during primate evolution. J Allergy Clin Immunol 2008;121(5):1262-18.

17. Trivedi NN, Tong Q, Raman K, et al. Mast cell alpha and beta tryptases changed rapidly during primate speciation and evolved from gamma-like transmembrane peptidases in ancestral vertebrates. J Immunol 2007;179(9):6072–9.

18. Wong GW, Foster PS, Yasuda S, et al. Biochemical and functional characterization of human transmembrane tryptase (TMT)/tryptase gamma. TMT is an exocytosed mast cell protease that induces airway hyperresponsiveness in vivo via an interleukin-13/interleukin-4 receptor alpha/signal transducer and activator of transcription (STAT) 6-dependent pathway. J Biol Chem 2002;277(44):41906–15.

19. Hansbro PM, Hamilton MJ, Fricker M, et al. Importance of mast cell Prss31/transmembrane tryptase/tryptase-γ in lung function and experimental chronic obstructive pulmonary disease and colitis. J Biol Chem 2014;289(26):18214–27.

20. Krishna MT, Chauhan A, Little L, et al. Inhibition of mast cell tryptase by inhaled APC 366 attenuates allergen-induced late-phase airway obstruction in asthma. J Allergy Clin Immunol 2001;107(6):1039–45.

21. Erin EM, Leaker BR, Zacharasiewicz A, et al. Effects of a reversible -tryptase and trypsin inhibitor (RWJ-58643) on nasal allergic responses. Clin Exp Allergy 2006; 36(4):458–64.

22. Giardina SF, Werner DS, Pingle M, et al. Novel, self-assembling dimeric inhibitors of human β tryptase. J Med Chem 2020;63(6):3004–27.

23. Elrod KC, Moore WR, Abraham WM, et al. Lactoferrin, a potent tryptase inhibitor, abolishes late-phase airway responses in allergic sheep. Am J Respir Crit Care Med 1997;156(2 Pt 1):375–81.

24. Hallgren J, Estrada S, Karlson U, et al. Heparin antagonists are potent inhibitors of mast cell tryptase. Biochemistry 2001;40(24):7342–9.

25. Rymut SM, Sukumaran S, Sperinde G, et al. Dose-dependent inactivation of airway tryptase with a novel dissociating anti-tryptase antibody (MTPS9579A) in healthy participants: a randomized trial. Clin Trans Sci 2022;15(2):451–63.

26. Tremaine WJ, Brezezinski A, Katz JA, et al. Treatment of mildly to moderately active ulcerative colitis with a tryptase inhibitor (APC 2059): an open-label pilot study. Aliment Pharmacol Ther 2002;16(3):407–13.

27. Yoshida N, Isozaki Y, Takagi T, et al. Review article: anti-tryptase therapy in inflammatory bowel disease. Aliment Pharmacol Ther 2006;24(Suppl 4):249–55.

28. Mori S, Itoh Y, Shinohata R, et al. Nafamostat mesilate is an extremely potent inhibitor of human tryptase. J Pharm Sci 2003;92(4):420–3.

29. Nimishakavi S, Raymond WW, Gruenert DC, et al. Divergent inhibitor susceptibility among airway lumen-accessible tryptic proteases. PLoS One 2015;10(10): e0141169.

30. Akula S, Fu Z, Wernersson S, et al. The evolutionary history of the chymase locus -a locus encoding several of the major hematopoietic serine proteases. Int J Mol Sci 2021;22(20):10975.

31. Kanefendt F, Thuss U, Becka M, et al. Pharmacokinetics, safety, and tolerability of the novel chymase inhibitor BAY 1142524 in healthy male volunteers. Clin Pharmacol Drug Dev 2019;8(4):467–79.

32. Duengen HD, Kober L, Nodari S, et al. Safety and tolerability of the chymase inhibitor fulacimstat in patients with left ventricular dysfunction after myocardial infarction-results of the CHIARA MIA 1 trial. Clin Pharmacol Drug Dev 2019; 8(7):942–51.

33. Duengen HD, Kim RJ, Zahger D, et al. Effects of the chymase inhibitor fulacimstat on adverse cardiac remodeling after acute myocardial infarction–results of the Chymase Inhibitor in Adverse Remodeling after Myocardial Infarction (CHIARA MIA) 2 trial. Am Heart J 2020;224:129–37.

34. Rossing P, Strand J, Avogaro A, et al. Effects of the chymase inhibitor fulacimstat in diabetic kidney disease–results from the CADA DIA trial. Nephrol Dial Transplant 2021;36(12):2263–73.

35. Hof P, Mayr I, Huber R, et al. The 1.8 Å crystal structure of human cathepsin G in complex with Suc-Val-Pro-PheP-(OPh)2: a Janus-faced proteinase with two opposite specificities. EMBO J 1996;15(20):5481–91.

36. Raymond WW, Trivedi NN, Makarova A, et al. How immune peptidases change specificity: cathepsin G gained tryptic function but lost efficiency during primate evolution. J Immunol 2010;185(9):5360–8.

37. Raymond WW, Su S, Makarova A, et al. Alpha 2-macroglobulin capture allows detection of mast cell chymase in serum and creates a reservoir of angiotensin II-generating activity. J Immunol 2009;182(9):5770–7.

38. Schechter NM, Irani AM, Sprows JL, et al. Identification of a cathepsin G-like proteinase in the MCTC type of human mast cell. J Immunol 1990;145(8):2652–61.

39. Maryanoff BE, de Garavilla L, Greco MN, et al. Dual inhibition of cathepsin G and chymase is effective in animal models of pulmonary inflammation. Am J Respir Crit Care Med 2010;181(3):247–53.

40. Miller BE, Mayer RJ, Goyal N, et al. Epithelial desquamation observed in a phase I study of an oral cathepsin C inhibitor (GSK2793660). Br J Clin Pharmacol 2017; 83(12):2813–20.

41. Toomes C, James J, Wood AJ, et al. Loss-of-function mutations in the cathepsin C gene result in periodontal disease and palmoplantar keratosis. Nat Genet 1999; 23(4):421–4.

42. Chalmers JD, Haworth CS, Metersky ML, et al. Phase 2 trial of the DPP-1 inhibitor brensocatib in bronchiectasis. N Engl J Med 2020;383(22):2127–37.

43. Wolters PJ, Muilenburg D, Pham CT, et al. Dipeptidyl peptidase I is essential for in vivo activation of mast cell chymases, but not tryptases, in mice. J Biol Chem 2001;276(21):18551–6.

44. Le QT, Gomez G, Zhao W, et al. Processing of human protryptase in mast cells involves cathepsins L, B, and C. J Immunol 2011;187(4):1912–8.

45. Caughey GH, Zerweck EH, Vanderslice P. Structure, chromosomal assignment, and deduced amino acid sequence of a human gene for mast cell chymase. J Biol Chem 1991;266(20):12956–63.

46. Reynolds DS, Gurley DS, Stevens RL, et al. Cloning of cDNAs that encode human mast cell carboxypeptidase A, and comparison of the protein with mouse mast cell carboxypeptidase A and rat pancreatic carboxypeptidases. Proc Natl Acad Sci USA 1989;86(23):9480–4.

47. Natsuaki M, Stewart CB, Vanderslice P, et al. Human skin mast cell carboxypeptidase: functional characterization, cDNA cloning, and genealogy. J Invest Dermatol 1992;99(2):138–45.

48. Akula S, Hellman L, Aviles FX, et al. Analysis of the mast cell expressed carboxypeptidase A3 and its structural and evolutionary relationship to other vertebrate carboxypeptidases. Dev Comp Immunol 2022;127:104273.

49. Tanco S, Lorenzo J, Garcia-Pardo J, et al. Proteome-derived peptide libraries to study the substrate specificity profiles of carboxypeptidases. Mol Cell Proteomics 2013;12(8):2096–110.

50. Kokkonen JO, Vartiainen M, Kovanen PT. Low density lipoprotein degradation by secretory granules of rat mast cells. Sequential degradation of apolipoprotein B by granule chymase and carboxypeptidase A. J Biol Chem 1986;261(34): 16067–72.
51. Lundequist A, Tchougounova E, Abrink M, et al. Cooperation between mast cell carboxypeptidase A and the chymase mouse mast cell protease 4 in the formation and degradation of angiotensin II. J Biol Chem 2004;279(31):32339–44.
52. Irani AM, Goldstein SM, Wintroub BU, et al. Human mast cell carboxypeptidase. Selective localization to MCTC cells. J Immunol 1991;147(1):247–53.
53. Goldstein SM, Leong J, Schwartz LB, et al. Protease composition of exocytosed human skin mast cell protease-proteoglycan complexes. Tryptase resides in a complex distinct from chymase and carboxypeptidase. J Immunol 1992;148(8): 2475–82.
54. Schneider LA, Schlenner SM, Feyerabend TB, et al. Molecular mechanism of mast cell-mediated innate defense against endothelin and snake venom sarafotoxin. J Exp Med 2007;204(11):2629–39.
55. Magnusdottir EI, Grujic M, Bergman J, et al. Mouse connective tissue mast cell proteases tryptase and carboxypeptidase A3 play protective roles in itch induced by endothelin-1. J Neuroinflammation 2020;17(1):123.
56. Dougherty RH, Sidhu SS, Raman K, et al. Accumulation of intraepithelial mast cells with a unique protease phenotype in T(H)2-high asthma. J Allergy Clin Immunol 2010;125(5):1046–53.
57. Takabayashi T, Kato A, Peters AT, et al. Glandular mast cells with distinct phenotype are highly elevated in chronic rhinosinusitis with nasal polyps. J Allergy Clin Immunol 2012;130(2):410–20.
58. Siddhuraj P, Clausson CM, Sanden C, et al. Lung mast cells have a high constitutive expression of carboxypeptidase A3 mRNA that is independent from granule-stored CPA3. Cells 2021;10(2):309.
59. Fricker M, Gibson PG, Powell H, et al. A sputum 6-gene signature predicts future exacerbations of poorly controlled asthma. J Allergy Clin Immunol 2019;144(1): 51–60.
60. Feyerabend TB, Weiser A, Tietz A, et al. Cre-mediated cell ablation contests mast cell contribution in models of antibody- and T cell-mediated autoimmunity. Immunity 2011;35(5):832–44.

UNITED STATES POSTAL SERVICE®

Statement of Ownership, Management, and Circulation
(All Periodicals Publications Except Requester Publications)

1. Publication Title	2. Publication Number	3. Filing Date
IMMUNOLOGY AND ALLERGY CLINICS OF NORTH AMERICA	006 – 361	9/18/2023

4. Issue Frequency	5. Number of Issues Published Annually	6. Annual Subscription Price
FEB, MAY, AUG, NOV	4	$365.00

7. Complete Mailing Address of Known Office of Publication (Not printer) (Street, city, county, state, and ZIP+4®)

ELSEVIER INC.
230 Park Avenue, Suite 800
New York, NY 10169

Contact Person
Malathi Samayan

Telephone (Include area code)
91-44-4299-4507

8. Complete Mailing Address of Headquarters or General Business Office of Publisher (Not printer)

ELSEVIER INC.
230 Park Avenue, Suite 800
New York, NY 10169

9. Full Names and Complete Mailing Addresses of Publisher, Editor, and Managing Editor (Do not leave blank)

Publisher (Name and complete mailing address)

Dolores Meloni, ELSEVIER INC.
1600 JOHN F KENNEDY BLVD. SUITE 1600
PHILADELPHIA, PA 19103-2899

Editor (Name and complete mailing address)

TAYLOR HAYES, ELSEVIER INC.
1600 JOHN F KENNEDY BLVD. SUITE 1600
PHILADELPHIA, PA 19103-2899

Managing Editor (Name and complete mailing address)

PATRICK MANLEY, ELSEVIER INC.
1600 JOHN F KENNEDY BLVD. SUITE 1600
PHILADELPHIA, PA 19103-2899

10. Owner (Do not leave blank. If the publication is owned by a corporation, give the name and address of the corporation immediately followed by the names and addresses of all stockholders owning or holding 1 percent or more of the total amount of stock. If not owned by a corporation, give the names and addresses of the individual owners. If owned by a partnership or other unincorporated firm, give its name and address as well as those of each individual owner. If the publication is published by a nonprofit organization, give its name and address.)

Full Name	Complete Mailing Address
WHOLLY OWNED SUBSIDIARY OF REED/ELSEVIER, US HOLDINGS	1600 JOHN F KENNEDY BLVD. SUITE 1600 PHILADELPHIA, PA 19103-2899

11. Known Bondholders, Mortgagees, and Other Security Holders Owning or Holding 1 Percent or More of Total Amount of Bonds, Mortgages, or Other Securities. If none, check box ► ☐ None

Full Name	Complete Mailing Address
N/A	

12. Tax Status (For completion by nonprofit organizations authorized to mail at nonprofit rates) (Check one)
The purpose, function, and nonprofit status of this organization and the exempt status for federal income tax purposes:
☒ Has Not Changed During Preceding 12 Months
☐ Has Changed During Preceding 12 Months (Publisher must submit explanation of change with this statement)

PS Form **3526**, July 2014 [Page 1 of 4 (see instructions page 4)] PSN: 7530-01-000-9931   PRIVACY NOTICE: See our privacy policy on www.usps.com.

---

13. Publication Title		14. Issue Date for Circulation Data Below
IMMUNOLOGY AND ALLERGY CLINICS OF NORTH AMERICA		AUGUST 2023

15. Extent and Nature of Circulation			Average No. Copies Each Issue During Preceding 12 Months	No. Copies of Single Issue Published Nearest to Filing Date
a. Total Number of Copies (Net press run)			102	92
b. Paid Circulation (By Mail and Outside the Mail)	(1)	Mailed Outside-County Paid Subscriptions Stated on PS Form 3541 (Include paid distribution above nominal rate, advertiser's proof copies, and exchange copies)	69	60
	(2)	Mailed In-County Paid Subscriptions Stated on PS Form 3541 (Include paid distribution above nominal rate, advertiser's proof copies, and exchange copies)	0	0
	(3)	Paid Distribution Outside the Mails Including Sales Through Dealers and Carriers, Street Vendors, Counter Sales, and Other Paid Distribution Outside USPS®	17	13
	(4)	Paid Distribution by Other Classes of Mail Through the USPS (e.g. First-Class Mail®)	14	17
c. Total Paid Distribution (Sum of 15b (1), (2), (3), and (4))			100	90
d. Free or Nominal Rate Distribution (By Mail and Outside the Mail)	(1)	Free or Nominal Rate Outside-County Copies included on PS Form 3541	1	1
	(2)	Free or Nominal Rate In-County Copies Included on PS Form 3541	0	0
	(3)	Free or Nominal Rate Copies Mailed at Other Classes Through the USPS (e.g. First-Class Mail)	0	0
	(4)	Free or Nominal Rate Distribution Outside the Mail (Carriers or other means)	1	1
e. Total Free or Nominal Rate Distribution (Sum of 15d (1), (2), (3) and (4))			2	2
f. Total Distribution (Sum of 15c and 15e)			102	92
g. Copies not Distributed (See Instructions to Publishers #4 (page #3))			0	0
h. Total (Sum of 15f and g)			102	92
i. Percent Paid (15c divided by 15f times 100)			98.04%	97.83%

* If you are claiming electronic copies, go to line 16 on page 3. If you are not claiming electronic copies, skip to line 17 on page 3.

16. Electronic Copy Circulation		Average No. Copies Each Issue During Preceding 12 Months	No. Copies of Single Issue Published Nearest to Filing Date
a. Paid Electronic Copies	►		
b. Total Paid Print Copies (Line 15c) + Paid Electronic Copies (Line 16a)	►		
c. Total Print Distribution (Line 15f) + Paid Electronic Copies (Line 16a)	►		
d. Percent Paid (Both Print & Electronic Copies) (16b divided by 16c × 100)	►		

☒ I certify that 50% of all my distributed copies (electronic and print) are paid above a nominal price.

17. Publication of Statement of Ownership

☒ If the publication is a general publication, publication of this statement is required. Will be printed
in the NOVEMBER 2023 issue of this publication.   ☐ Publication not required.

18. Signature and Title of Editor, Publisher, Business Manager, or Owner		Date
Malathi Samayan - Distribution Controller	*Malathi Samayan*	9/18/2023

I certify that all information furnished on this form is true and complete. I understand that anyone who furnishes false or misleading information on this form or who omits material or information requested on the form may be subject to criminal sanctions (including fines and imprisonment) and/or civil sanctions (including civil penalties).

PS Form **3526**, July 2014 (Page 3 of 4)   PRIVACY NOTICE: See our privacy policy on www.usps.com

Moving?

Make sure your subscription moves with you!

To notify us of your new address, find your **Clinics Account Number** (located on your mailing label above your name), and contact customer service at:

Email: journalscustomerservice-usa@elsevier.com

800-654-2452 (subscribers in the U.S. & Canada)
314-447-8871 (subscribers outside of the U.S. & Canada)

Fax number: 314-447-8029

Elsevier Health Sciences Division
Subscription Customer Service
3251 Riverport Lane
Maryland Heights, MO 63043

*To ensure uninterrupted delivery of your subscription, please notify us at least 4 weeks in advance of move.

Printed and bound by CPI Group (UK) Ltd, Croydon, CR0 4YY

03/10/2024

01040474-0018